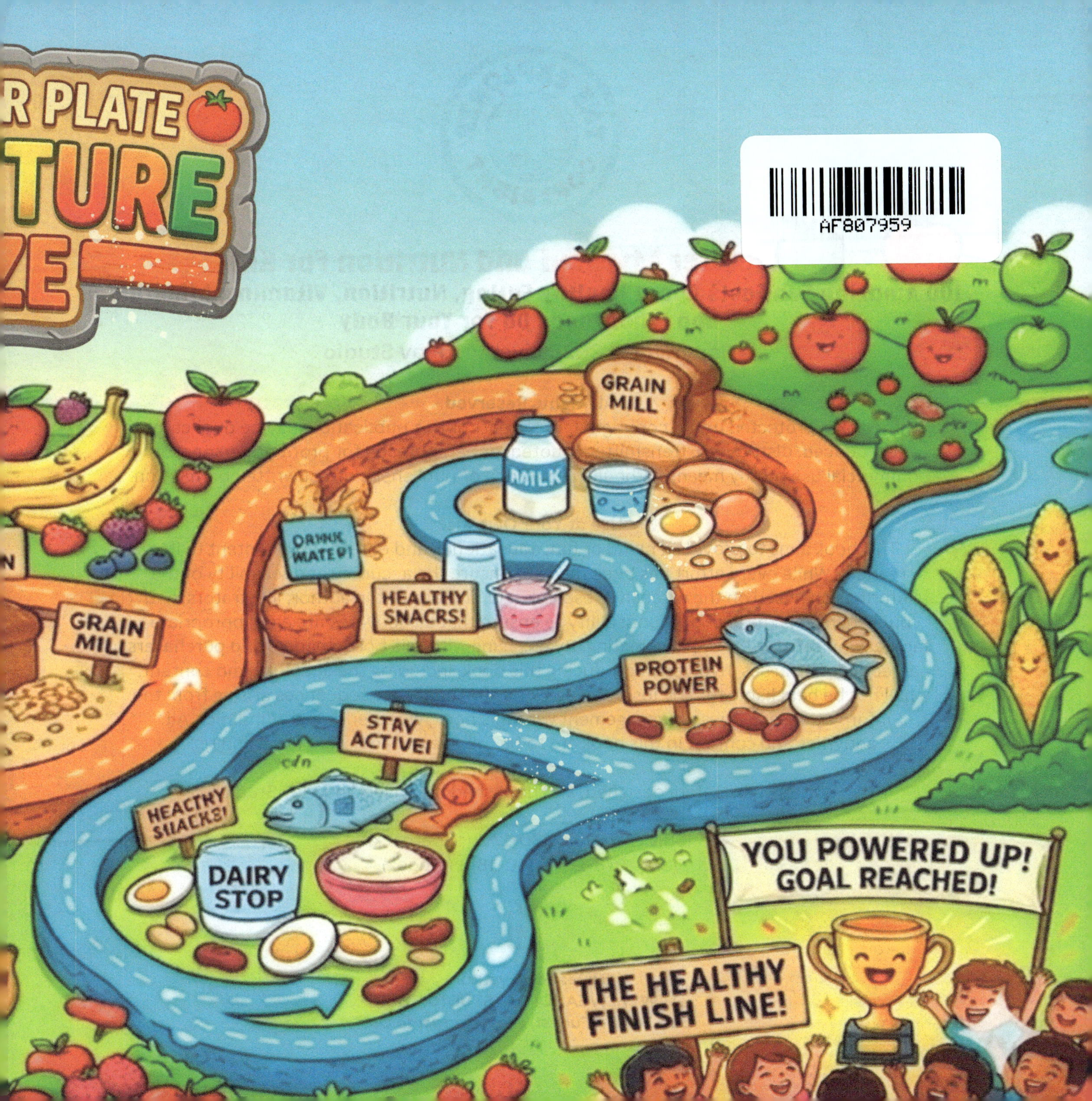
R PLATE
TURE
ZE
GRAIN MILL
MILK
HEALTHY SNACRS!
PROTEIN POWER
STAY ACTIVE!
GRAIN MILL
DAIRY STOP
YOU POWERED UP! GOAL REACHED!
THE HEALTHY FINISH LINE!

The Explorer My Food and Nutrition for Kids

100 Amazing Fun Facts About Healthy Eating, Nutrition, Vitamins, Minerals, and What Foods Do for Your Body

Use at Your Own Risk

This book aims to provide a blend of fun, educational, and entertaining content to its readers. While every effort has been made to ensure the accuracy and reliability of the information based on the extensive research and findings of the author, illustrators, and publishers, it is the user's responsibility to ensure that all activities are age-appropriate, factual, and safe for those participating. By engaging with this book, readers and purchasers agree that all parties involved in producing this book, including the activities and content, shall not be held liable for any loss, damage, or unfortunate consequences arising from the information, activities, or engagement with this book, whether direct or indirect. All activities and content in this book are to be followed at your discretion and risk.

Written, illustrated, designed, and published by © Live And Play Studio

ISBN: 978-1-963130-17-1 (paperback)
ISBN: 978-1-963130-18-8 (e-book)

@liveandplaystudio
WWW.LIVEANDPLAYSTUDIO.COM
Live To The Fullest, Play Alongside Us.

HELLOO!!

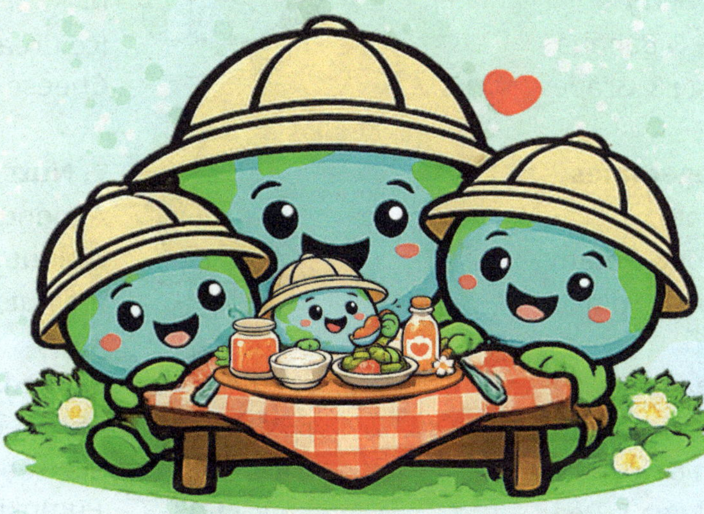

A Note to Parents

Thank you for choosing The Explorer My Foods & Nutrients. This book is designed to spark curiosity and provide children with introductory knowledge about a selective variety of foods in a fun, engaging way. This book is for entertainment and general education only. Since dietary needs differ, please consult a health or nutrition professional for personal advice.

We hope this book brings joy and discovery to your child's learning.

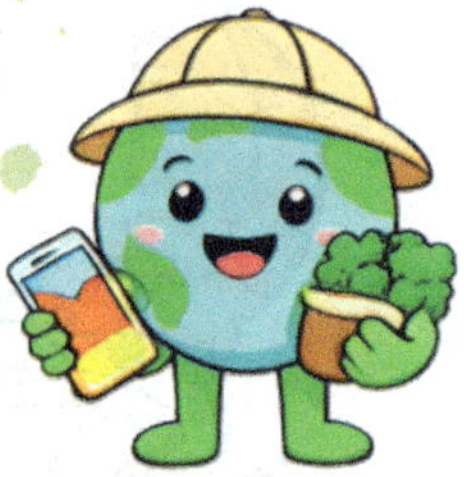
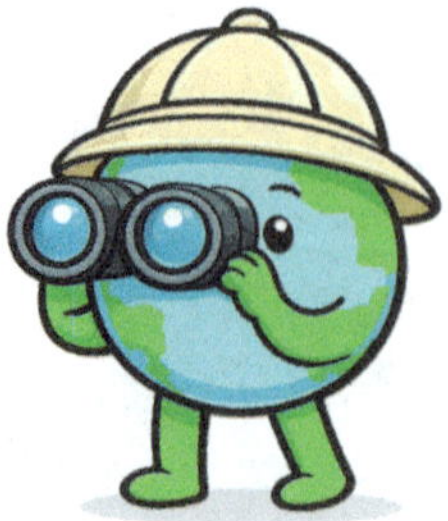

Table of Contents

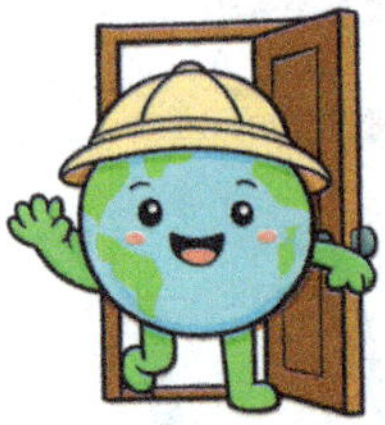

Sneak Inside
Healthy Vitamins Wheel
The Rainbow Color Foods

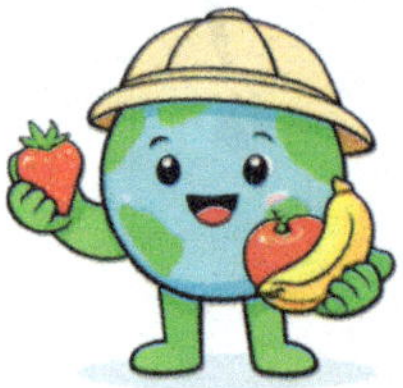

1. Fruits
Strawberry
Apple & Banana
Orange & Grapes

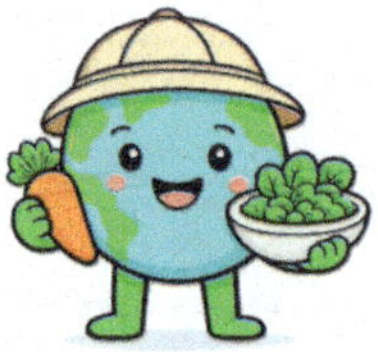

2. Vegetables
Tomato
Carrot & Potato
Onion & Spinach

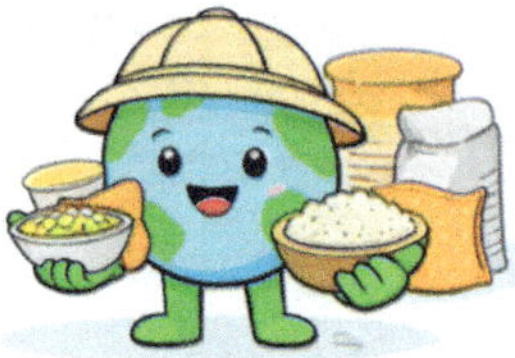

3. Legumes
Peanut
Bean & Soybean
Chickpea & Pea

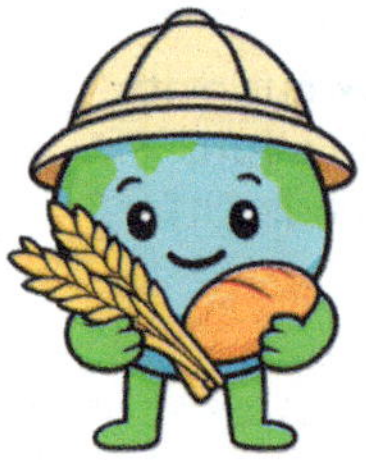

4. Whole Grains
Whole Wheat
Oat & Brown Rice
Quinoa & Barley

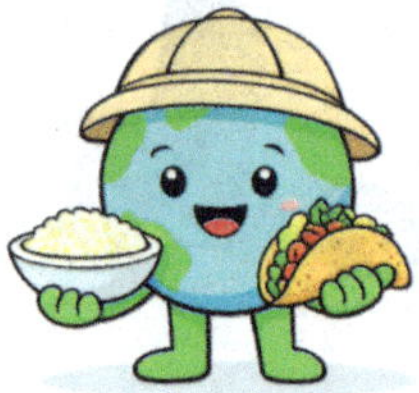

5. Refined Grains
Pasta
White Bread & White Rice
Flour Tortilla & Couscous

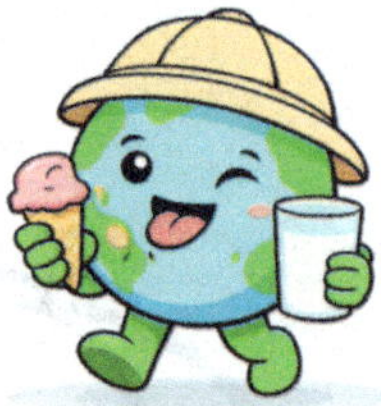

6. Dairy
Milk
Ice Cream & Butter
Cheese & Yogurt

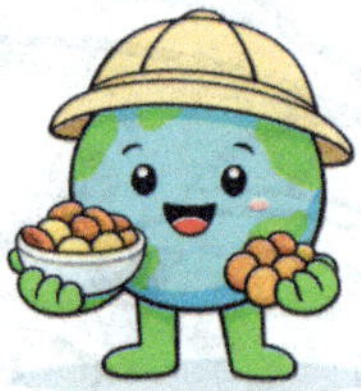

7. Nuts
Almond
Walnut & Cashew
Walnut & Pistachio

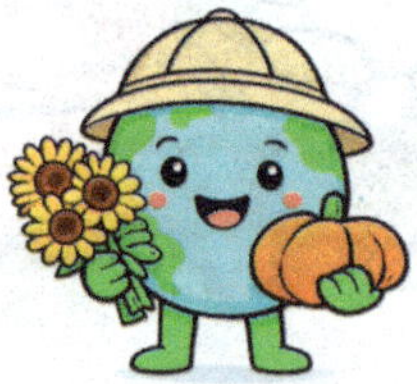

8. Seeds
Chia Seed
Flaxseed & Sunflower Seed
Pumpkin Seed & Sesame Seed

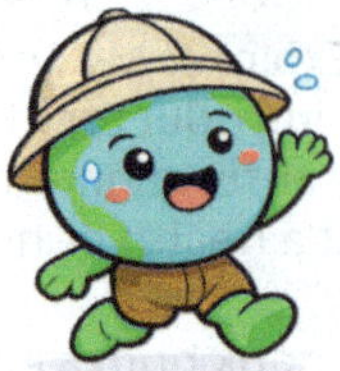

9. Poultry
Chicken
Turkey & Duck
Ostrich & Pheasant

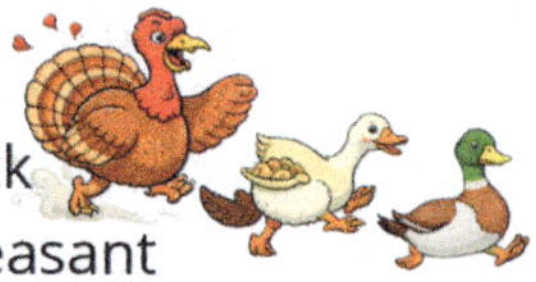

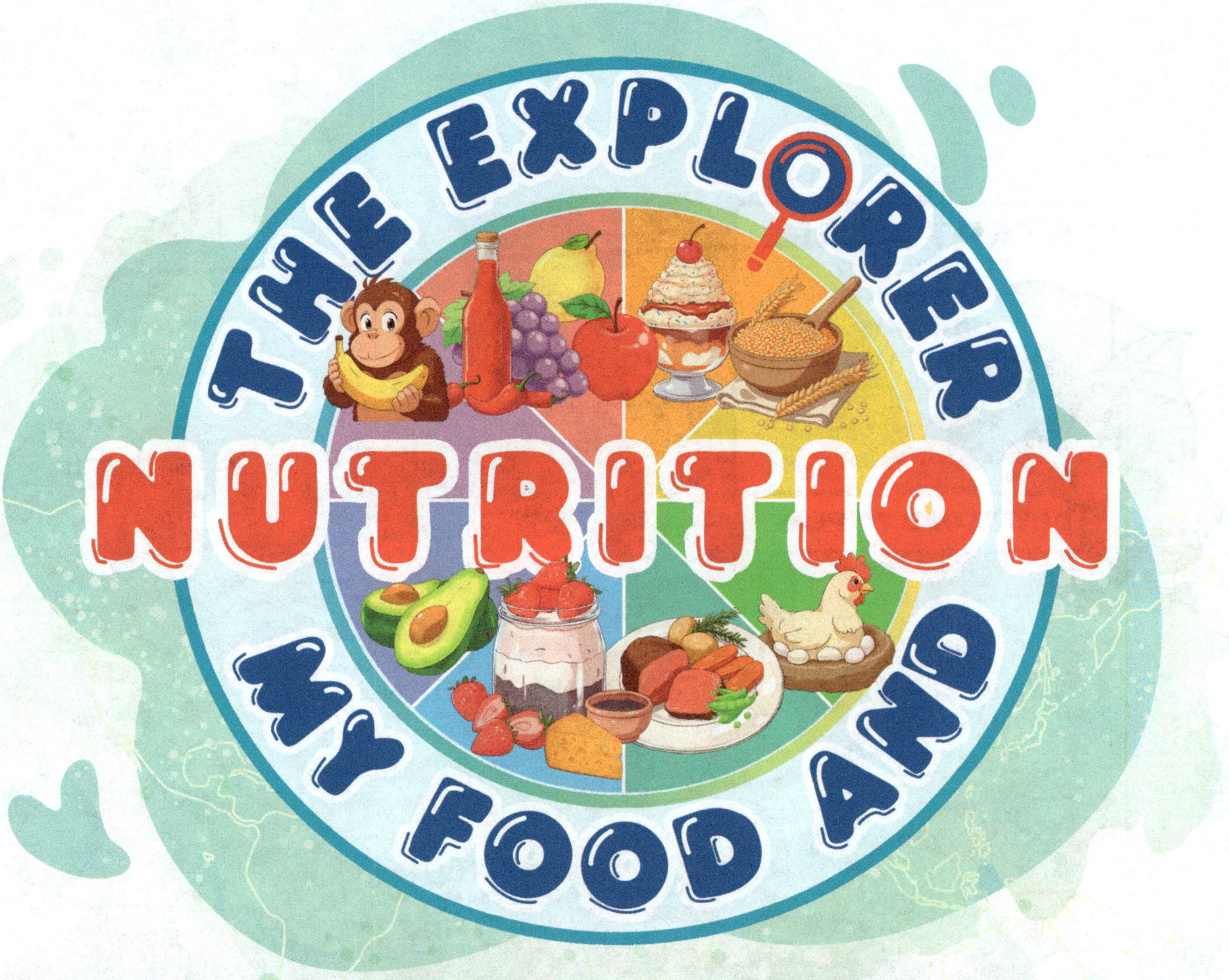

The Explorer My Food and Nutrition for Kids

100 Amazing Fun Facts About Healthy Eating, Nutrition, Vitamins, Minerals, and What Foods Do for Your Body

Live And Play Studio

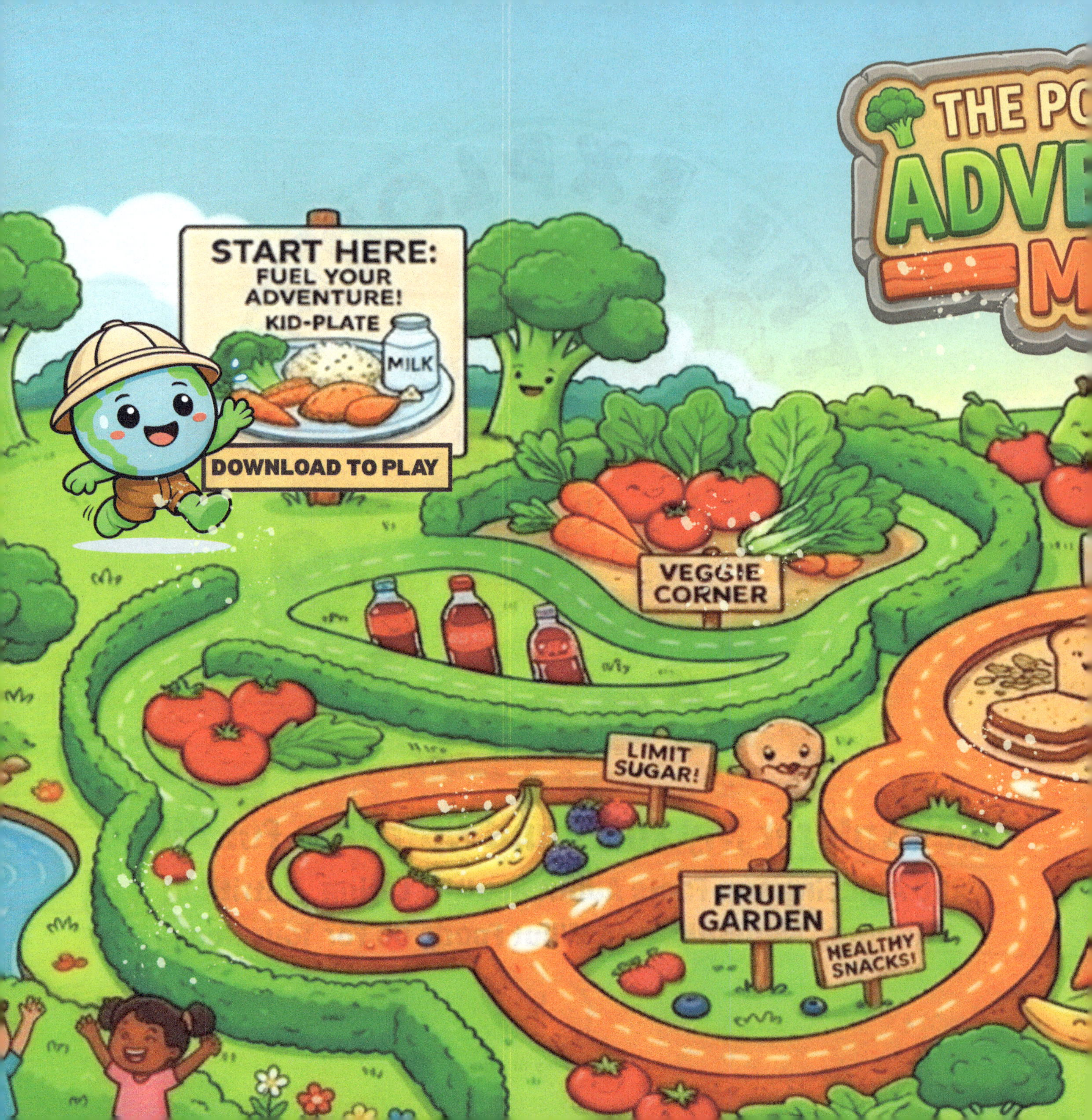
THE PO
ADVE
M
START HERE:
FUEL YOUR ADVENTURE!
KID-PLATE
MILK
DOWNLOAD TO PLAY
VEGGIE CORNER
LIMIT SUGAR!
FRUIT GARDEN
HEALTHY SNACKS!

EXPLORE INSIDE

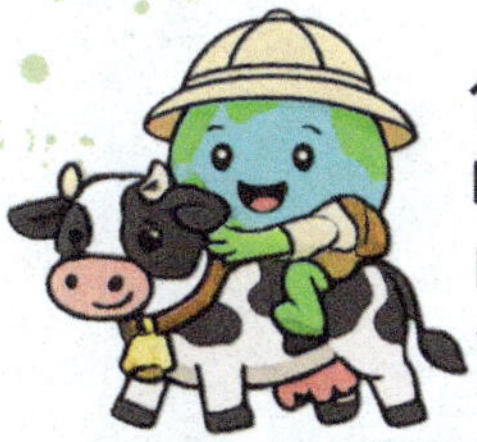

10. Red Meats
Beef
Pork & Lamb
Venison & Bison

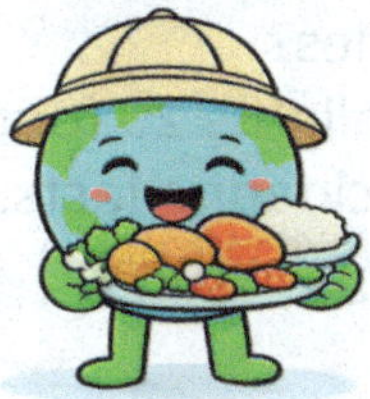

11. Offals or Organ Meats
Liver
Heart & Tripe
Tongue & Oxtail

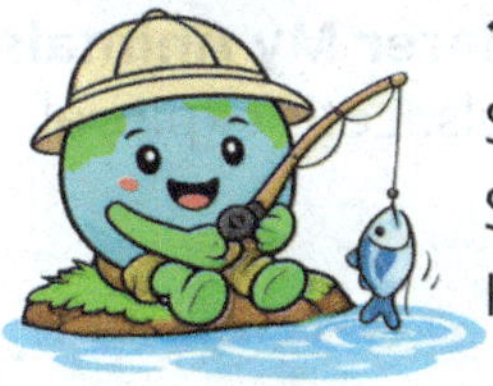

12. Fish
Salmon
Sardine & Tuna
Herring & Cod

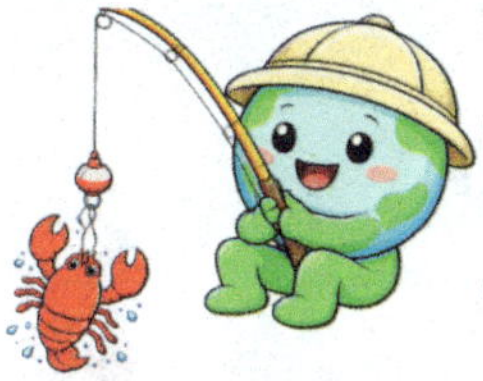

13. Shellfish
Oyster
Mussel & Shrimp
Crab & Lobster

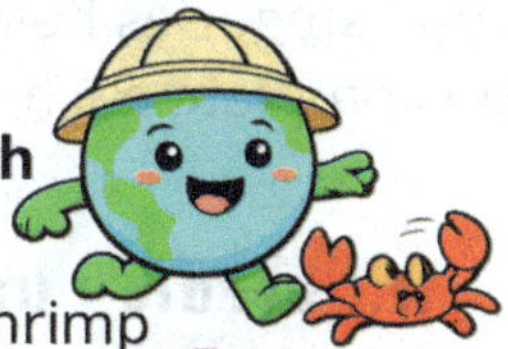

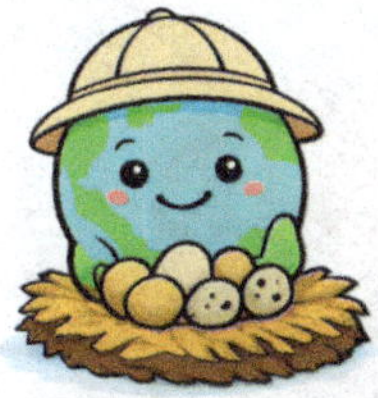

14. Eggs
Chicken Egg
Duck Egg & Quail Egg
Caviar & Roe

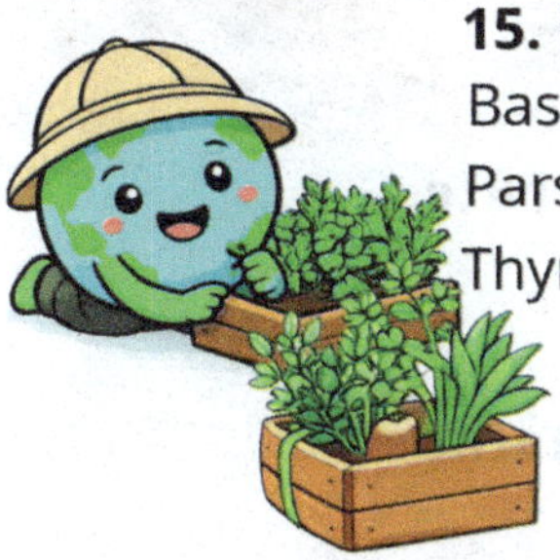

15. Herbs
Basil
Parsley & Rosemary
Thyme & Oregano

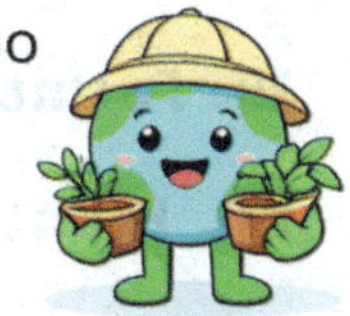

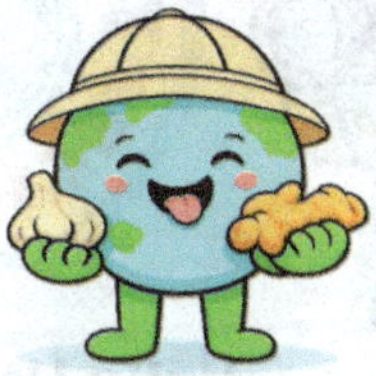

16. Spices
Garlic
Ginger & Turmeric
Pepper & Cinnamon

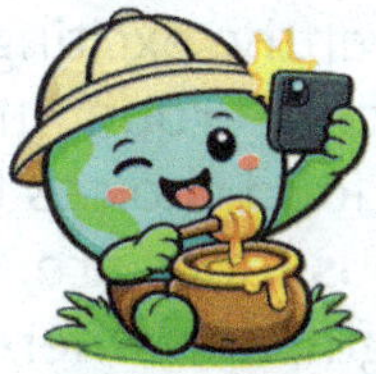

17. Natural Sugar
Sugarcane
Beet & Date
Maple & Honey

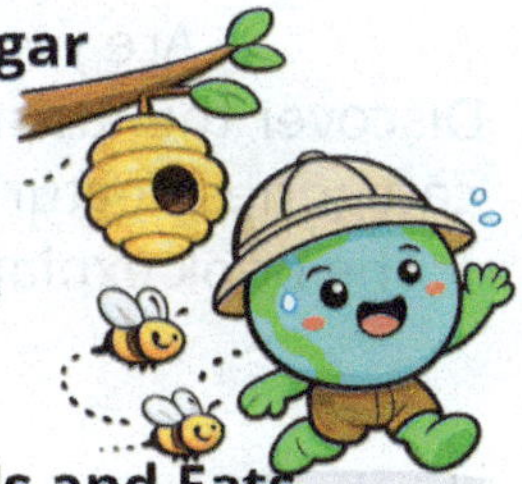

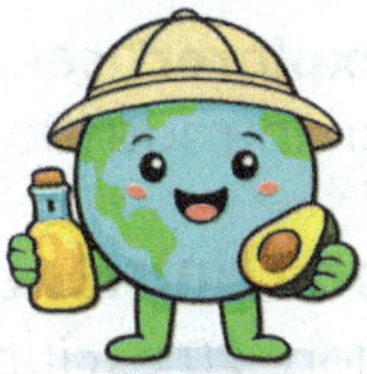

18. Healthy Oils and Fats
Olive
Avocado & Coconut Oil
Fish Oil & Ghee

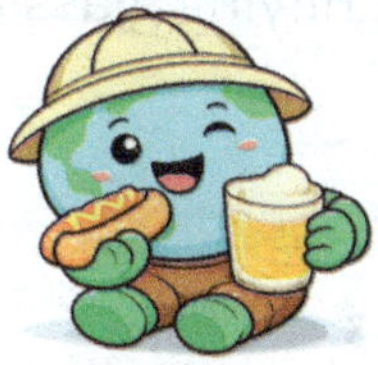

19. Fermented Foods
Sauerkraut
Kefir & Apple Cider
Kimchi & Miso

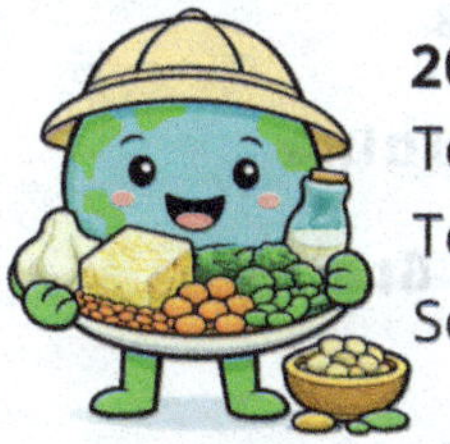

20. Plant-Based Proteins
Tofu
Tempeh & Edamame
Seitan & Lentil

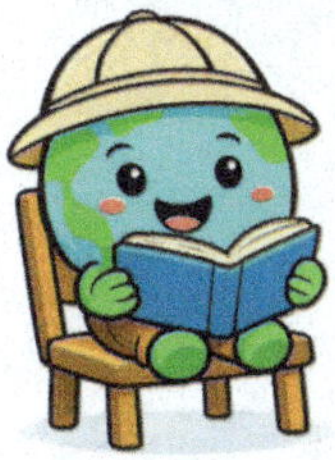

The Mouthful Words (Glossary)
The Explorer Fun Facts
Nutritional Value Guide
The Explorer Social
The Explorer Info
The Explorer Bonus

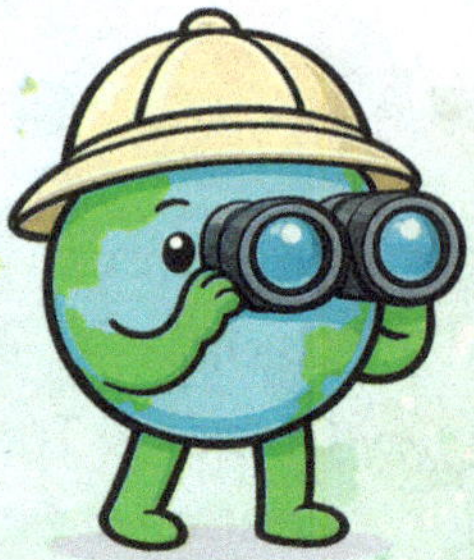

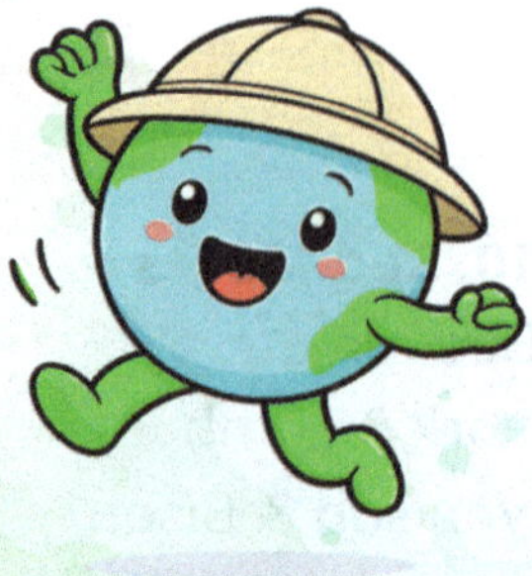

Hello Little Explorer!

Are you ready to discover the exciting benefits of a variety of food categories?
Discover the fascinating world of food around the world. This entertaining guide highlights 20 food categories, featuring 100 popular food choices from across the globe, along with fascinating facts. The book explains what nutritious foods are, how they help the body with energy, growth, and strength, and where these foods originate.

This book complements our **"The Explorer"** series, and more precisely, **"The Explorer My Animals Habitats,"** which offers readers an introduction to the captivating lives of animals. Let's explore!

The Food Nutrients And Their Benefits

Let's explore 20 exciting food categories below.
Check the magnifying glass as you complete each category.

1. Fruits
2. Vegetables
3. Legumes
4. Whole Grains
5. Refined Grains
6. Dairy
7. Nuts
8. Seeds
9. Poultry
10. Red Meats
11. Offals / Organ Meats
12. Fish
13. Shellfish
14. Eggs
15. Herbs
16. Spices
17. Spices
18. Healthy Oils and Fats
19. Fermented Foods
20. Plant-based Proteins

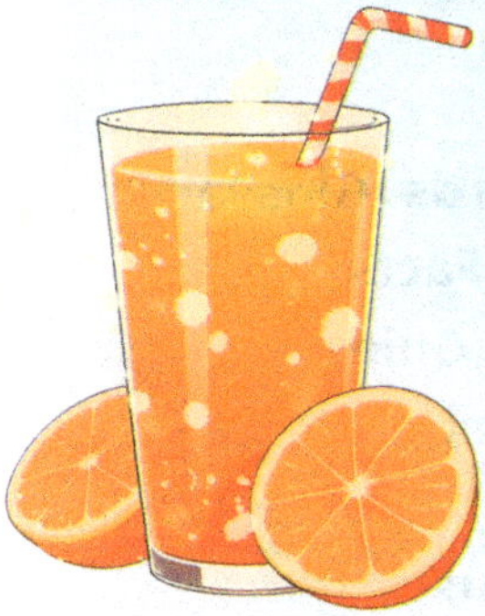

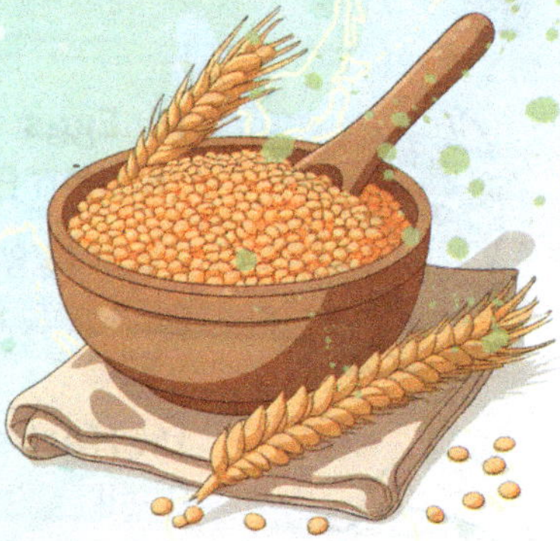

LET'S GO!!

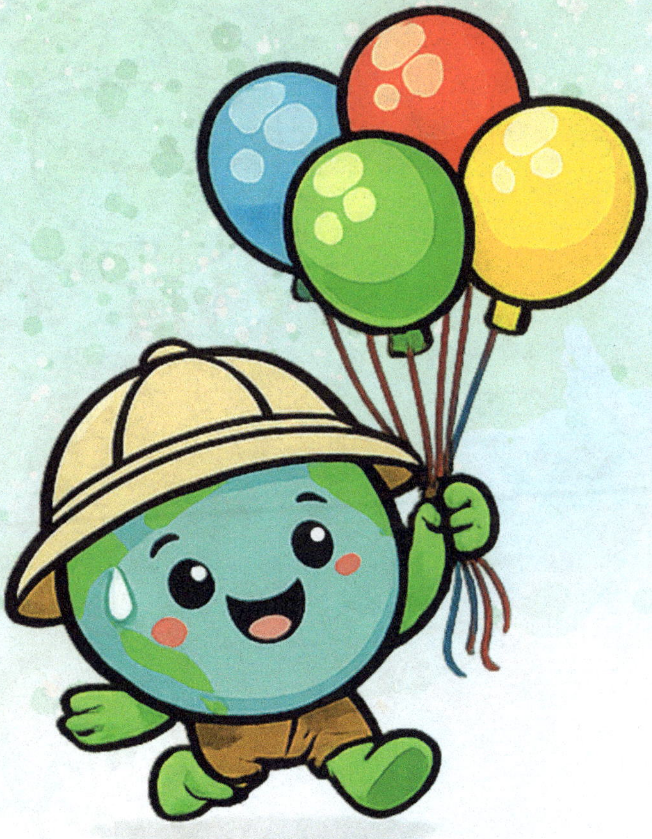

Healthy Vitamins

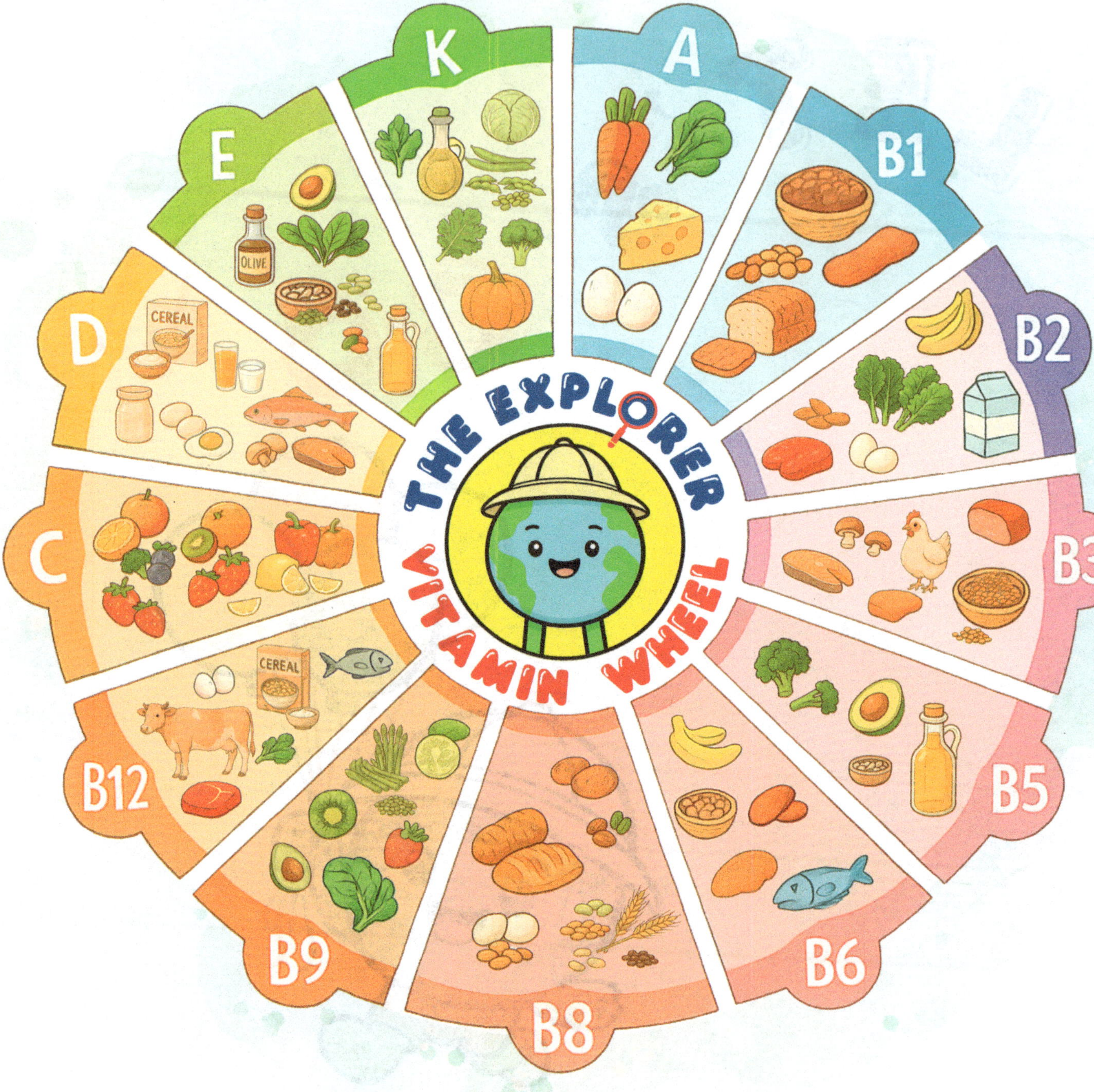

The Rainbow Color Foods

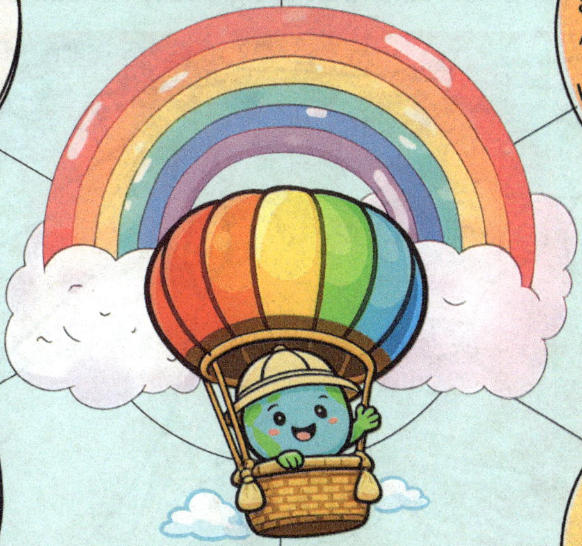

RED
Heart Health
Eating red foods can improve heart health and boost energy levels. They contain potent antioxidants that benefit the whole body.

ORANGE
Eye & Skin Health
Foods that are orange are full of natural vitamin A, which improves vision, supports heart health, boosts energy, and promotes healthy skin.

YELLOW
Energy & Happiness
Yellow foods bring a sunny glow to your health! With vitamin C and healthy carbs, it provides a boost of energy and improves mood.

GREEN
Growth & Detox
Green foods help your body grow strong and tall. They flush out toxins, support healthy gut bacteria, and leave you feeling fresh and active.

PURPLE
Brain Power
Purple foods boost memory and brain power. These foods are full of nutrients that support focus, learning, and improved problem-solving.

WHITE
Strong Immunity
White foods offer immune system support, shielding the body from germs, and helping you remain active.

1. Fruits

Fruits are naturally sweet, colorful, and nutritious. They contain important vitamins, minerals, fiber, and antioxidants that support a healthy immune system, help fight off sickness, and aid digestion. Apples, bananas, and oranges are examples of fruits cultivated on farms and orchards throughout tropical, temperate, and subtropical areas. Many fruits are harvested seasonally and transported globally, making them accessible year-round. Their natural flavor, variety, and convenience make fruits a popular food choice for snacks, juices, and desserts. Fruits are a healthy choice that helps support a balanced diet.

Isn't that a-fruit-some?

Now that you have been introduced to a fruit benefit, are you ready to discover some of the most popular fruits that are globally consumed

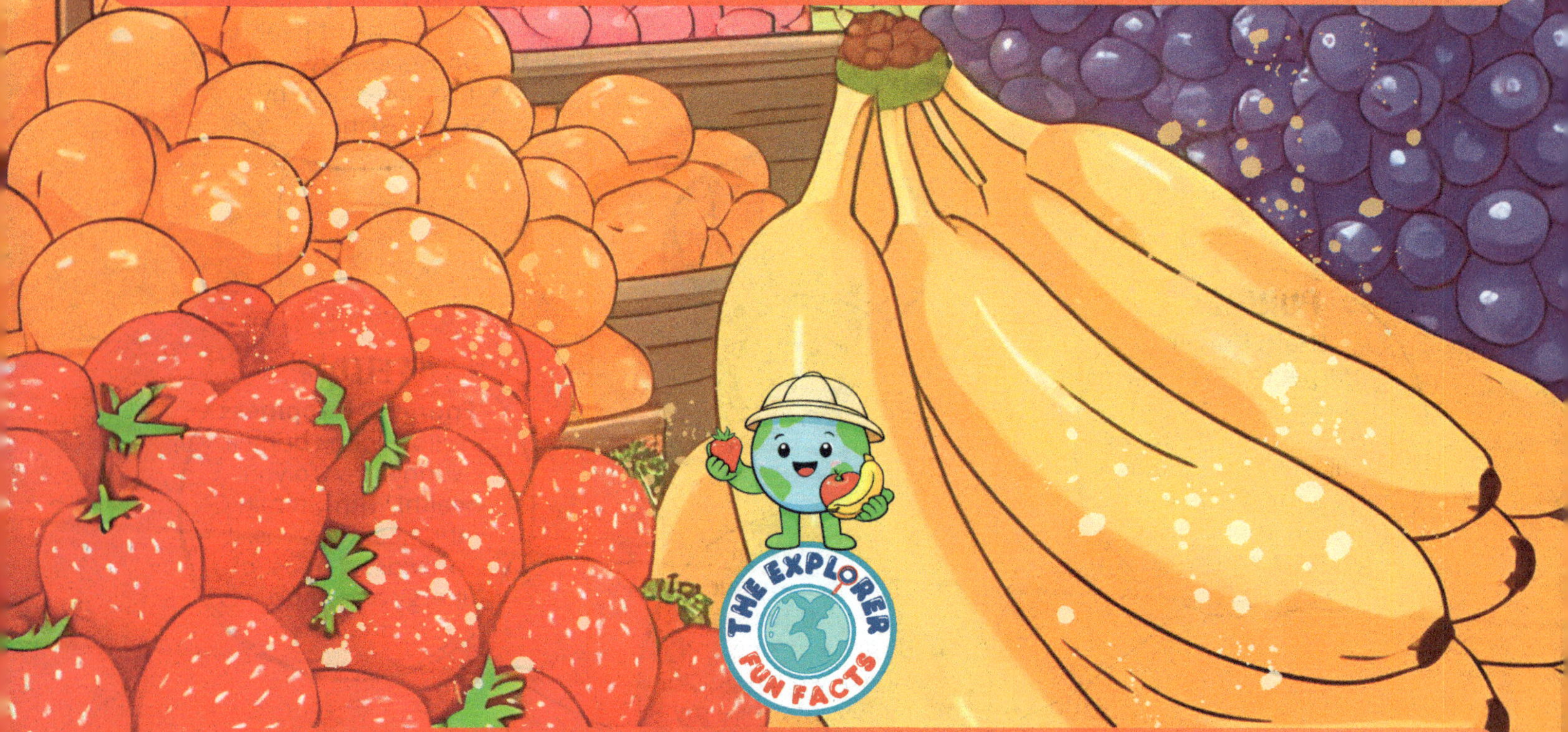

Do you know that pineapples don't grow on trees, but rather from the ground? Watermelons contain over 90% water, making them a refreshing and hydrating summer snack.

Strawberry

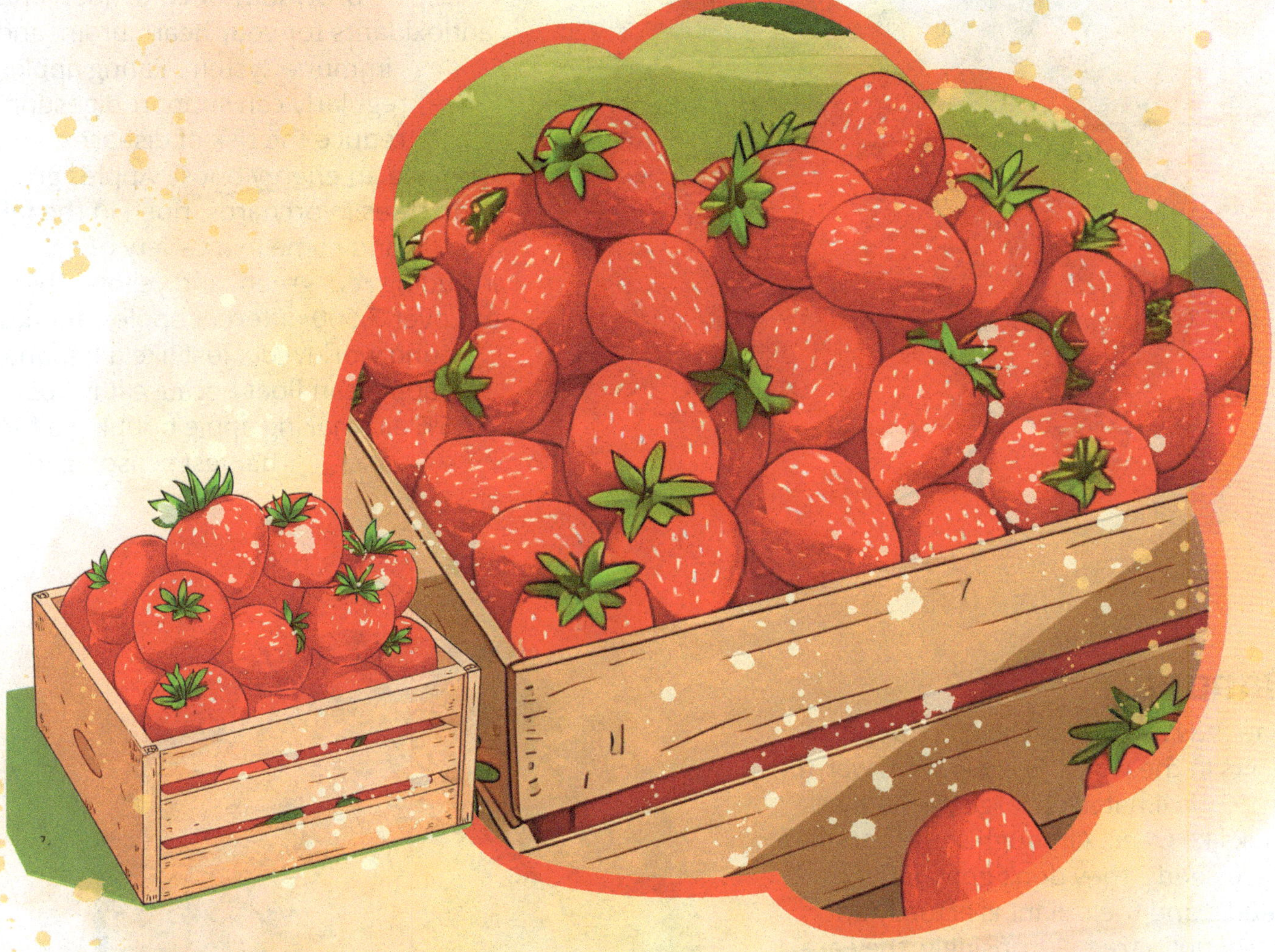

Strawberries are the stars of spring and Valentine's Day. They grow from small flowering plants in raised beds or potted containers. These heart-shaped, vibrant red, and juicy fruits are popular because of their sweetness and unique and enjoyable experience. Strawberries are technically not berries but belong to the rose family. It is the only fruit with seeds on the outside, with each fruit containing an average of 200 seeds. They are high in vitamin C, fiber, and antioxidants, which are beneficial for your skin, muscles, brain, and heart, and help reduce inflammation. Strawberries are great snacks or added to smoothies, desserts, and salads.
Do you know that the fear of strawberries is called Fragariaphobia?

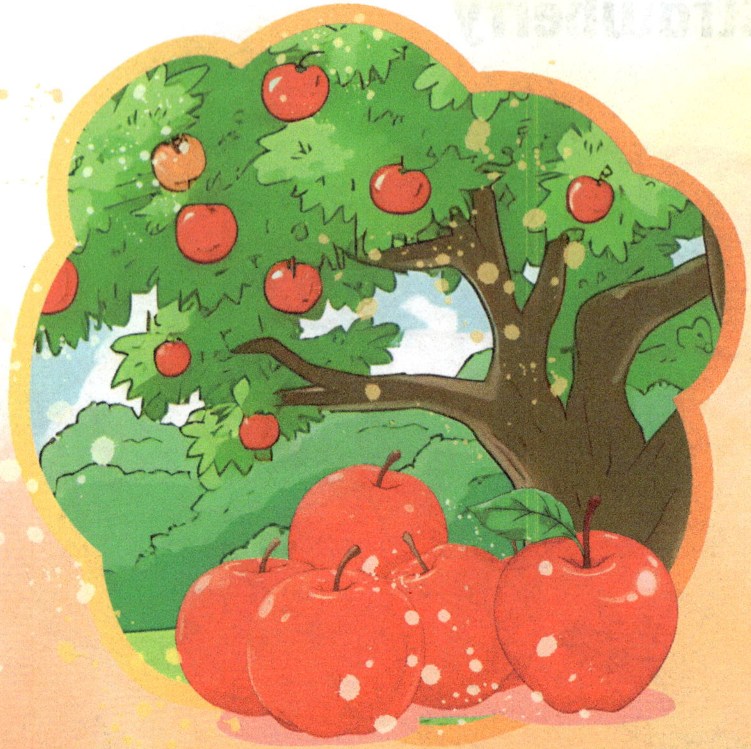

Apple

Apples are popular healthy fruits that provide vitamin C, fiber, and antioxidants for your heart, brain, and immune system. Eating apples regularly can support digestion, reduce the risk of diseases, and provide an energy boost. Apples grow on trees in orchards, ripen in the fall and come in a variety of colors, including red, green, and yellow. There are over 7,500 different apple varieties found worldwide. Just like a banana, an apple can float because it is about 25% air, making apple bobbing a fun harvest season game.

Banana

Bananas are one of the most popular fruits in the world. They grow in warm, tropical climates on large plants that look like trees. Although some bananas have seeds, they don't grow from seeds, and their plant is actually an herb, not a tree. Surprisingly, they are actually berries, but strawberries aren't. Bananas are a great source of potassium, which helps muscles work properly, and vitamin B6 is needed to support brain health. Did you know that bananas can also float in water just like apples?

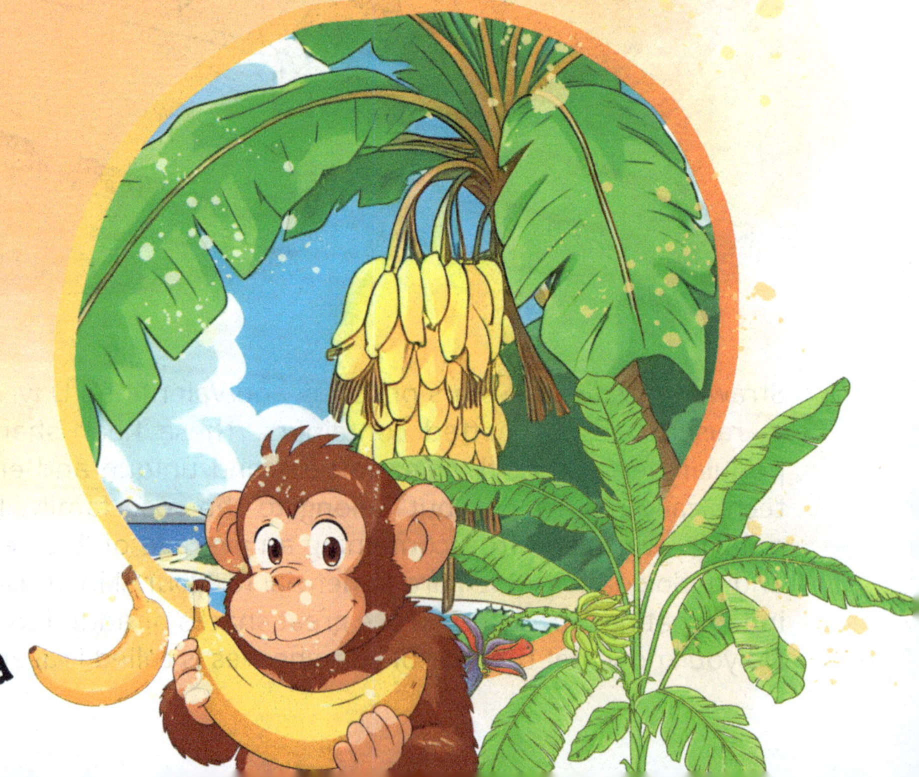

bananana

Orange

This vibrant, round, orange color fruit is remarkably juicy and thrives in warm climates, such as Florida, Spain, and Brazil. Oranges are fat-free and an excellent source of vitamin C, which helps boost iron absorption, strengthen the immune system to combat colds, and aid in wound healing. It also contains fiber, potassium, and antioxidants that keep your heart and skin healthy. You can consume an orange in various ways, and regardless, it provides more than your entire day's vitamin C. Some cultures consider oranges a symbol of good fortune and present them as gifts during New Year celebrations.

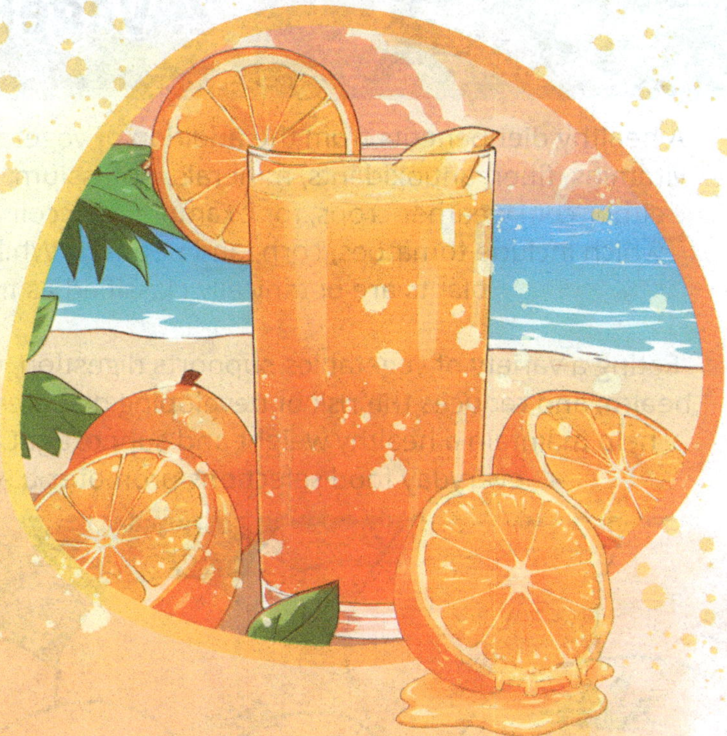

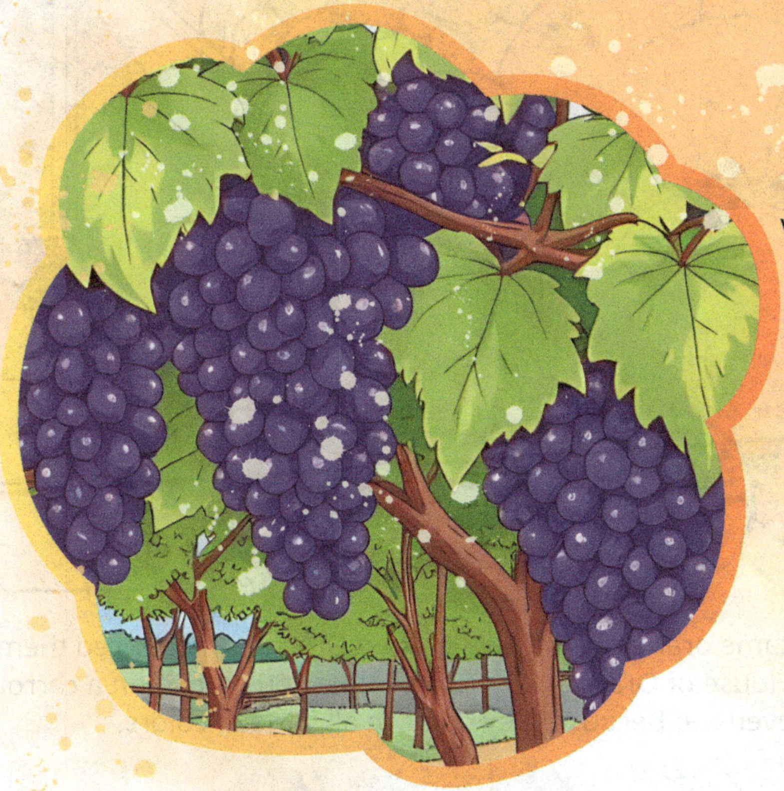

Grape

They come in red, green, and purple varieties and grow in clusters on vines, especially in sunny California, France, Italy, and Chile. Although grapes are small, they have lots of vitamin C, vitamin K, and calcium, which help keep your heart healthy, build strong bones, and prevent long-term diseases. Grapes contain a substance called resveratrol that promotes a healthy brain and can reduce the effects of cognitive decline. Dried grapes, also known as raisins, are a naturally sweet snack that provides a boost of energy.

2. Vegetables

A healthy diet benefits from the addition of vegetables, as they are sources of essential nutrients, vitamins, fiber, antioxidants, minerals, potassium, and magnesium. Vegetables are categorized as either cool weather crops, for example, broccoli, spinach, and carrots, or warm weather crops, which include tomatoes, corn, and peppers. While we often refer to them as vegetables, many plants are botanically classified as fruits because they contain seeds.

Eating a variety of vegetables supports digestion, enhances the immune system, promotes heart health, and reduces the risk of developing diabetes and cancer. Vegetables with high fiber content help maintain a healthy weight and support gut function. Including vibrant vegetables in your everyday food selections promotes a well-rounded nutrient consumption.

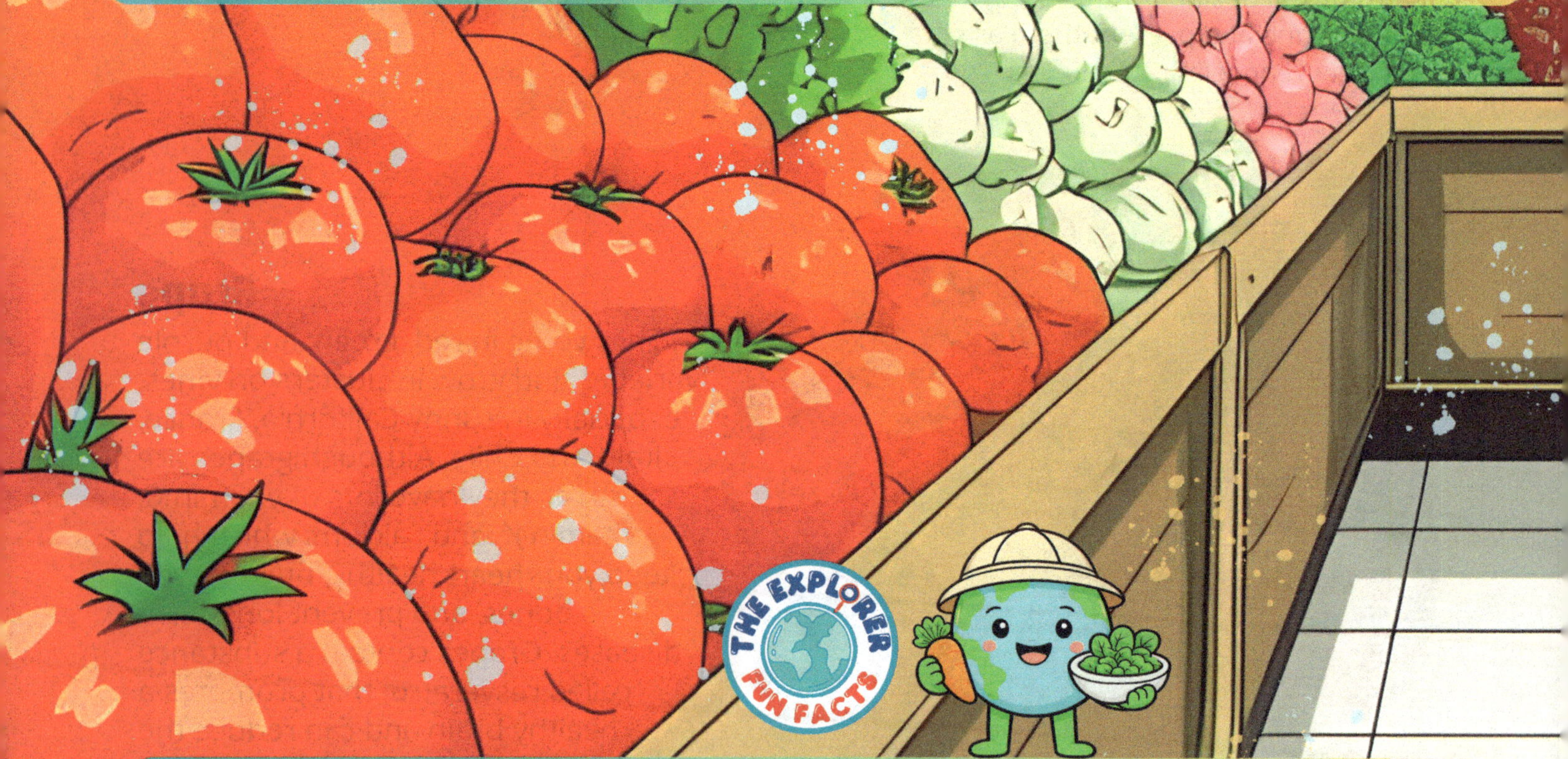

Carrots used to be purple. They only became orange in the 1600s when Dutch farmers bred them that way to honor their royal family, the House of Orange! So the next time you crunch on a carrot, imagine it in purple, yellow, or even red because they come in all sorts of colors.

Tomato

Tomatoes are juicy, with edible seeds and low in calories. Tomatoes are initially from the Andes region of South America and are a staple vegetable in the Mediterranean. It is rich in vitamin C and K, folate, potassium, and the powerful antioxidants that support heart health, protect against certain types of cancer, boost the immune system, and promote healthy skin. Tomatoes contain vitamin K, which is good for strong bones and helps prevent osteoporosis. Tomatoes can be eaten raw, cooked, or blended into sauces. It adds delicious flavor and color to ingredients such as spaghetti and pizza sauce. Its versatility has led NASA to cultivate tomatoes from seeds in a zero-gravity environment in space.

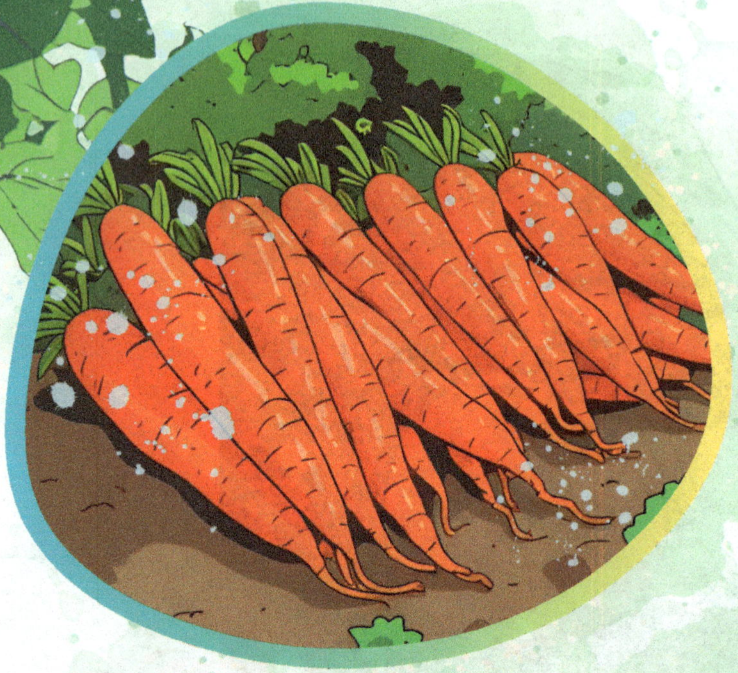

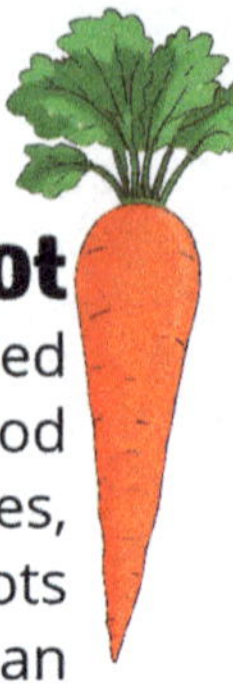

Carrot

This bright orange root vegetable is filled with vital nutrients that contribute to good health. It is delicious cooked in many dishes, great eaten raw, juiced, or blended. Carrots are naturally sweet, making them an appealing snack for children, adults, and animals alike. An excellent source of vitamins A and K1, fiber, antioxidants, and potassium that help maintain healthy vision, skin, and immune function. Adding carrots to your meals can help with digestion, lower the chances of long-term illnesses, and benefit your heart. They are a low-calorie, nutrient-dense food, perfect for healthy eating choices. It's not surprising that the rabbit loves it.

Potato

Did you know potatoes were the first vegetables grown in space in 1995? Potatoes are root vegetables and a source of complex carbohydrates, dietary fiber, potassium, vitamin B6, and vitamin C. It is low in calories, naturally gluten-free, and fat-free, providing lasting energy with no cholesterol or saturated fat when prepared without frying and with minimal heavy toppings. Potatoes are grown in North America, Europe, and Asia, with 4,000 different potato varieties that exist around the world. Potatoes are a nutritious and filling option for people of all ages, as they support muscle function and increase satiety when incorporated into a balanced diet.

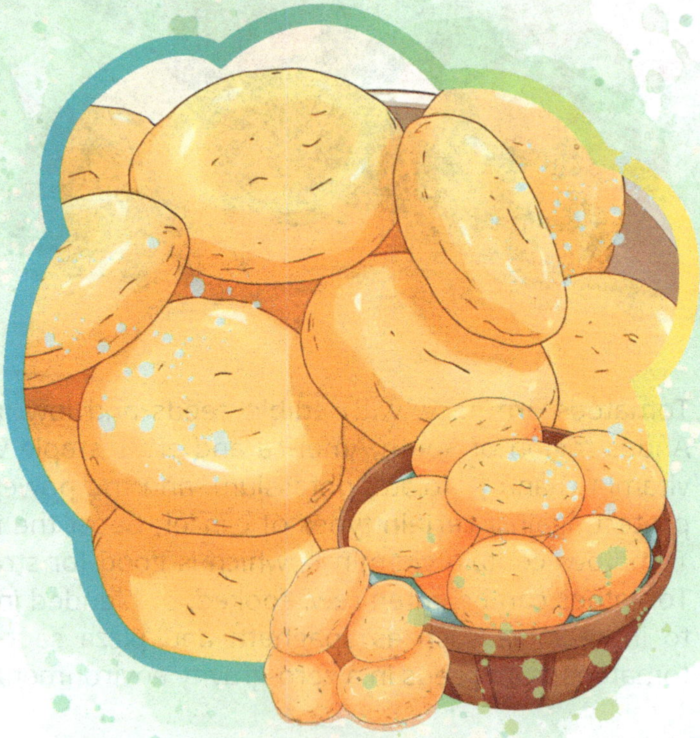

Onion

Onions are a flavorful bulb with a distinct taste, available in yellow, red, white, and green varieties. It is packed with antioxidants, high in vitamin C, and prebiotic fiber helps promote gut health, boost immunity, reduce inflammation, and regulate blood sugar levels. Onions enhance the flavor of food while also promoting health and preventing sickness. When you chop onions, they release fumes containing sulfur, which can make your eyes water and become irritated. However, chilling them first or cutting them underwater reduces the tears.

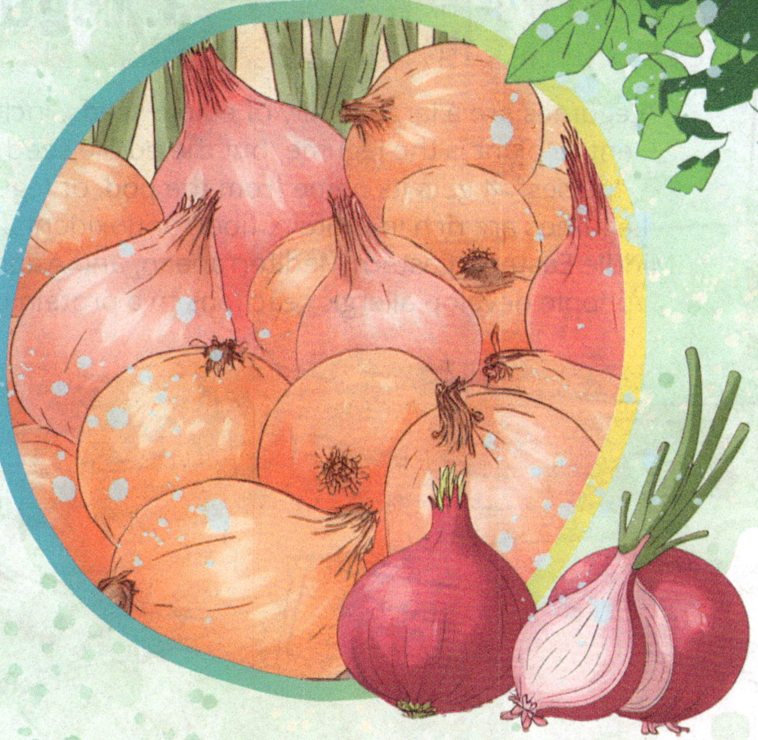

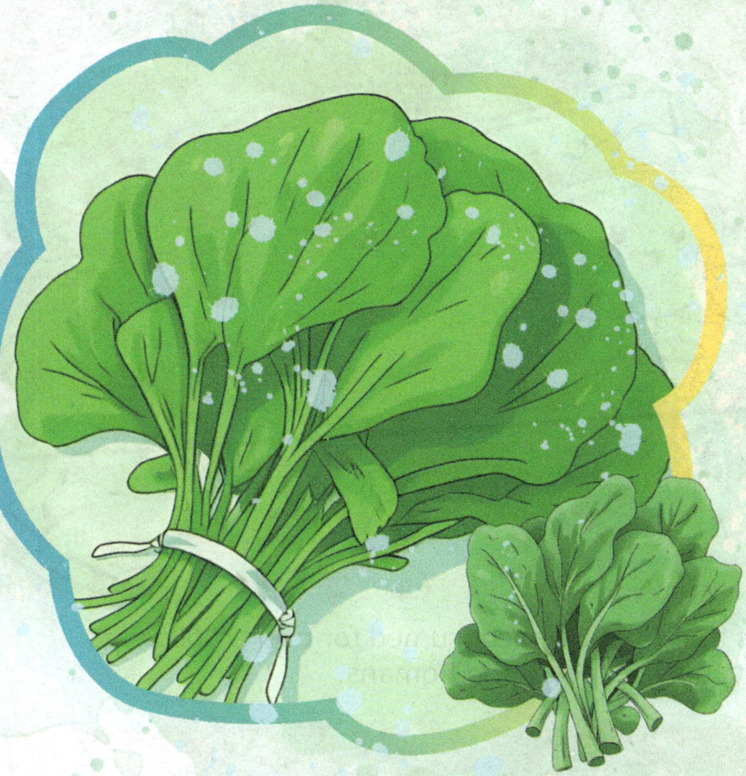

Spinach

Spinach is known for its richness in iron, vitamin K, vitamin A, folate, and magnesium, that are beneficial for healthy bones, boost immunity, and help create red blood cells. It's high in antioxidants that help fight inflammation and promote eye health. This leafy green vegetable is native to Central and Western Asia, and is enjoyed raw in salads, mixed into smoothies, or cooked in dishes. It gained its popularity due to the cartoon character Popeye, who ate it for immediate strength. Including spinach in your meals is a smart choice for boosting energy, growth, and overall wellness.

3. Legumes

Legumes are a large family of edible seeds, including peanuts, beans, lentils, and peas. The entire plant is the legume, but the edible seed inside legumes is typically dried and called "pulses". It gets its name from the pod, or legume, that protects the seeds as they ripen. Legumes are rich in protein, fiber, antioxidants, vitamins, and minerals. They are popular in Middle Eastern, Eastern Mediterranean, and Asian dishes. Despite its nutritional benefits, some people develop allergic reactions to a protein compound found in legumes called lectins.

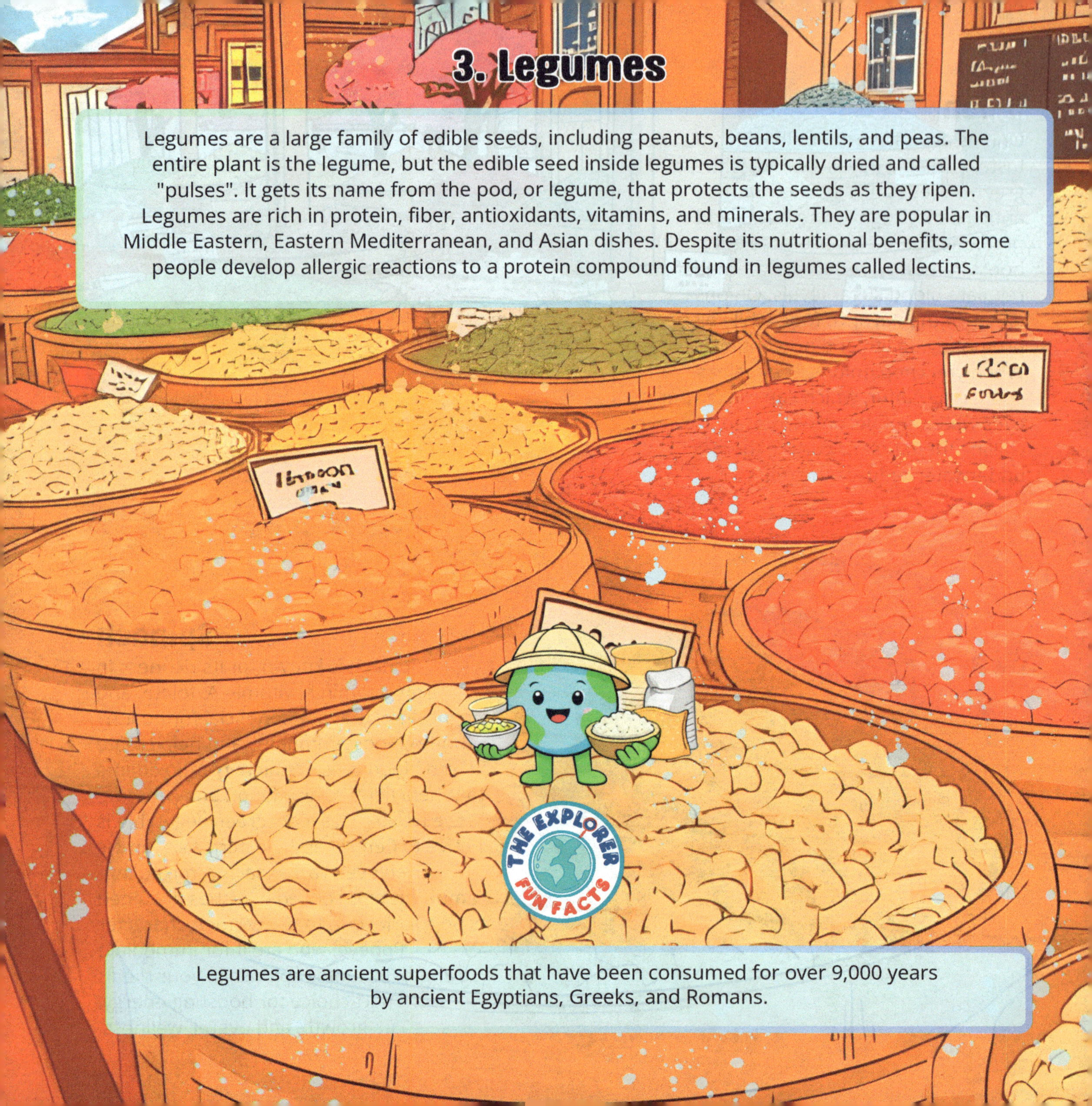

Legumes are ancient superfoods that have been consumed for over 9,000 years by ancient Egyptians, Greeks, and Romans.

Peanut

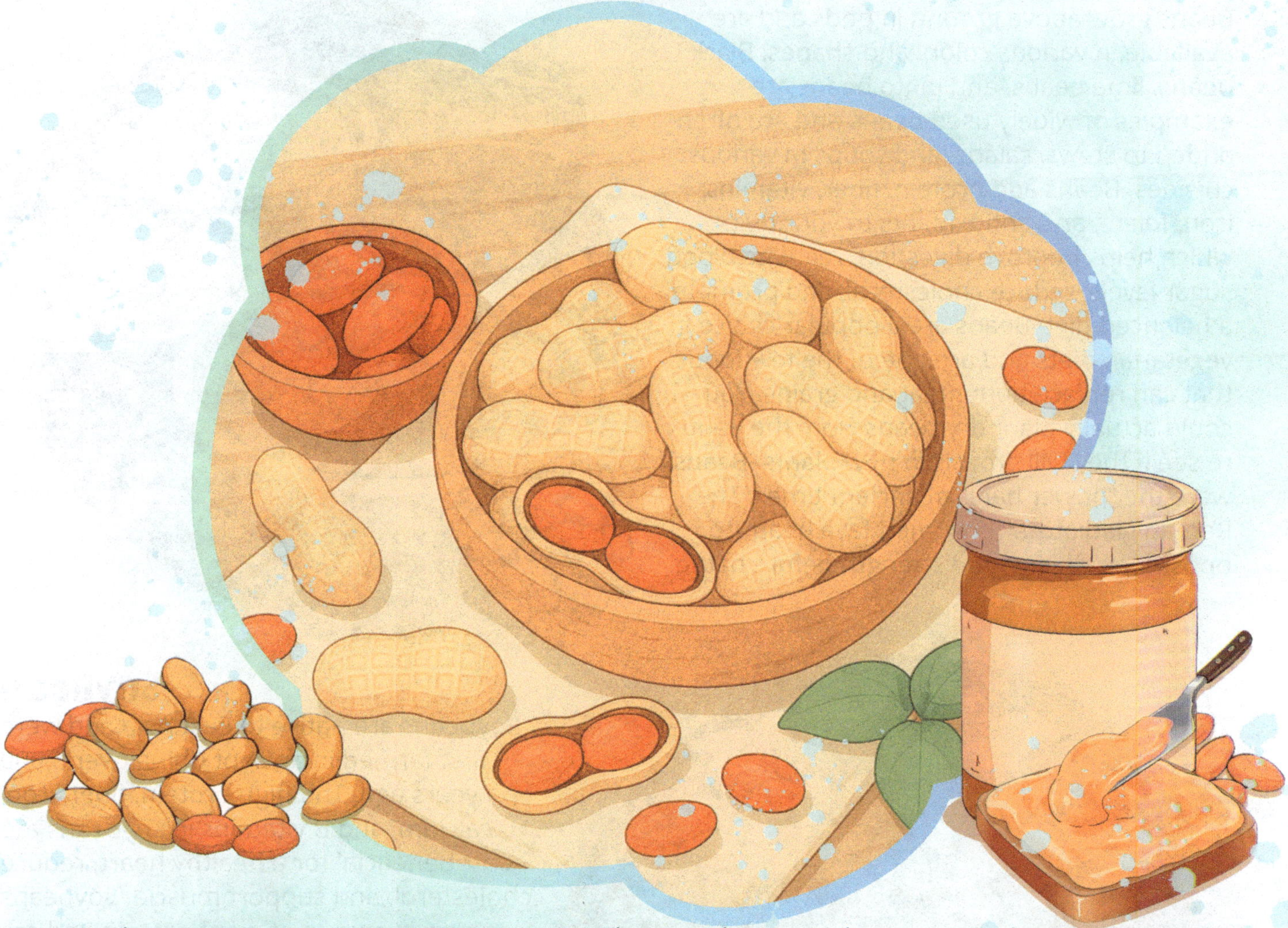

Despite their name, peanuts aren't true nuts. They are legumes that grow underground in pods related to beans and peas rather than tree nuts. Peanuts grow in tropical and subtropical climates of China, India, and the United States. They're nutrient-dense legumes packed with protein, healthy fats, fiber, vitamin E, niacin, and folate. Peanuts are rich in antioxidants, which support a healthy heart and may help reduce swelling. Vegetarians and health-conscious individuals will find these to be an excellent substitute for meat protein. Peanuts provide a feeling of fullness, lasting energy, and are often enjoyed in peanut butter and jelly sandwiches or as roasted snacks. No wonder our mom packed our bags with PBJ for our lunch. Adding peanuts to your meals may boost brain health, aid muscle recovery, and improve cholesterol levels. For optimal health, always select varieties that are unsalted and minimally processed. It takes over 500 peanuts in a 12-ounce jar of peanut butter. Their affordability makes them a smart, energy-boosting addition to daily nutrition.

Bean

Beans grow above ground in pods and are available in various colors and shapes. Black beans, lima beans, and pinto beans are examples of widely used beans and are often added to stews, salads, and soups in various cuisines. Beans add protein, fiber, vitamins, iron, folate, and antioxidants to your diet, which helps improve digestion, regulate blood sugar levels, reduce cholesterol, and promote a balanced diet. Beans are a popular choice in vegetarian diets and are one of the few foods that can replace both meat and grains. You could actually plant dry beans from the pantry to see if they will grow into new plants. Beans were the "power bars" of ancient times. The Roman gladiators consumed fava beans to boost their energy and strength before battle.

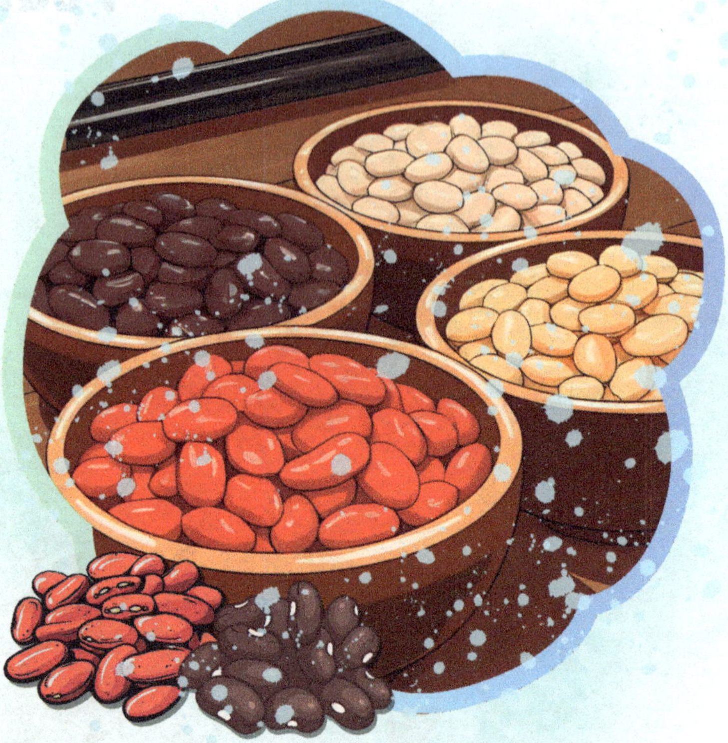

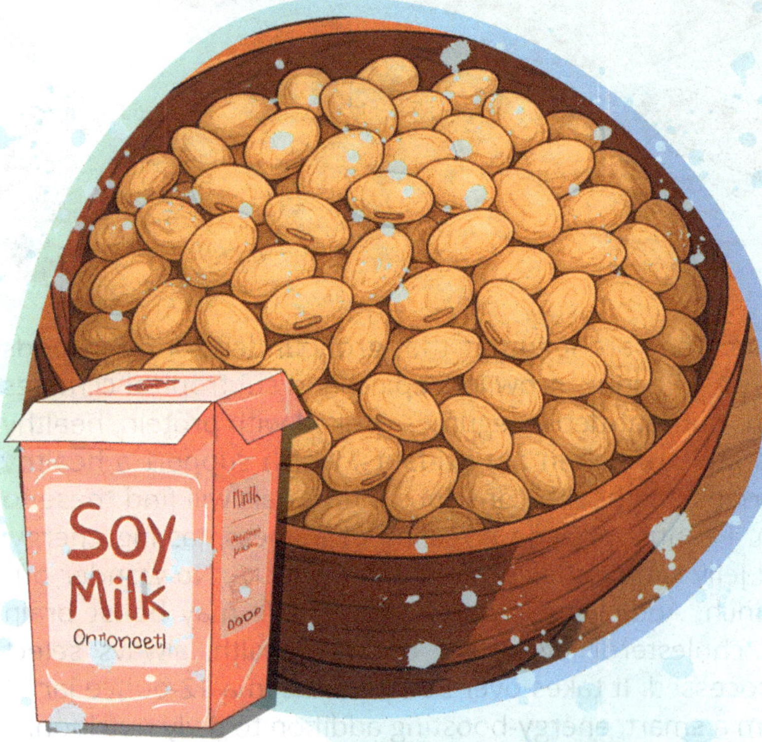

Soybean

Soybeans are native to East Asia and were first farmed in ancient China over 5,000 years ago. The high protein, fiber, iron, calcium, and B vitamins in soybeans are beneficial for a healthy heart, reduce cholesterol, and support muscle. Soybeans are a great source of plant protein and are commonly used to make foods such as tofu, soy milk, edamame, miso, and tempeh, which are ideal dairy substitutes for vegetarians and vegans. It contains isoflavones, natural compounds that may support bone health and hormonal balance. Similar to meat, soybeans are a rare plant-based food that provides a complete protein, containing all nine essential amino acids.

Chickpea

These beans, also known as garbanzo or Ceci beans, have been around for 7,500 years. Chickpeas are a staple in Middle Eastern, Mediterranean, and Indian cuisines to make dishes like hummus, stews, and salads. Due to their high protein, fiber, iron, and folate, they're a favored plant-based protein source for vegetarians and vegans. They support digestive health, help regulate blood sugar, and promote a healthy heart. Adding chickpeas to your diet provides essential energy to keep you full longer and supports a balanced eating habit. Chickpea plants possess a secret defense mechanism that releases a special acid from their leaves and stems, deterring insects.

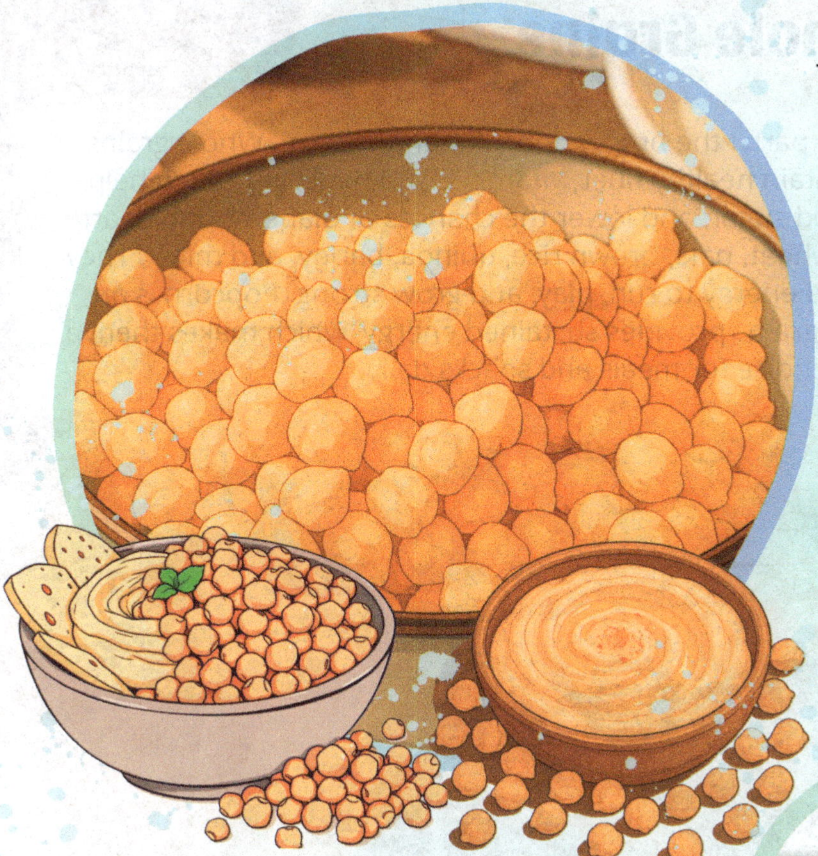

Pea

Peas have been grown in the Middle East for over 9,000 years. There are at least 37 varieties that have been cultivated since the Roman era. Their plants are natural climbers and can reach up to six feet tall. Among the favorites are snap peas and snow peas, loved for their crisp and edible pods. Peas are delicious raw or cooked in a simple side dish. Nutritionally, peas are packed with vitamins A, C, and K, fiber, protein, iron, and zinc. These nutrients are essential for increasing energy, strengthening the immune system, aiding digestion, and managing blood sugar levels.

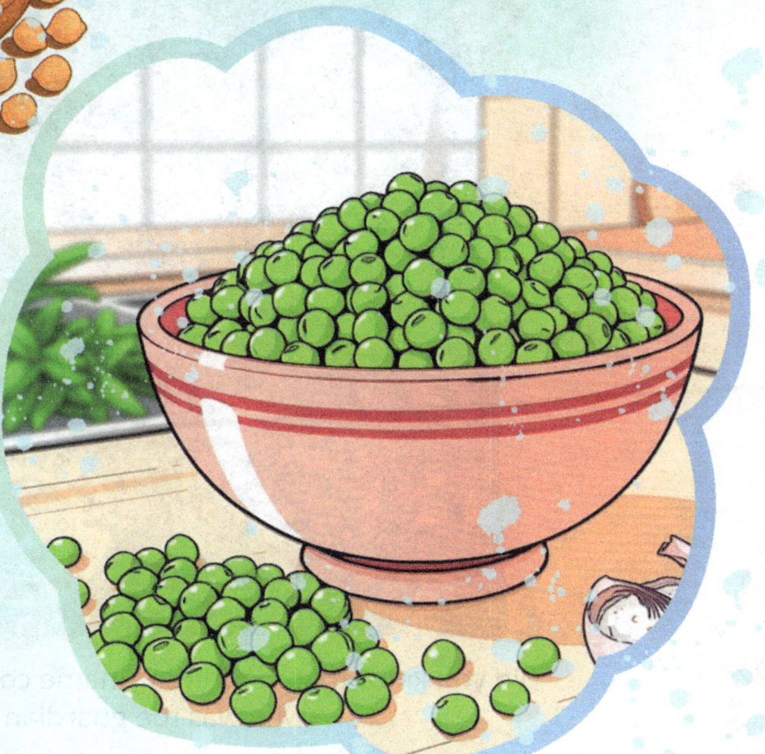

4. Whole Grains

Grains are the whole kernel that has three parts: the bran, germ, and endosperm. Whole grains are incredibly important because they contain healthy fiber, vitamins, and minerals, which help sustain energy, aid digestion, regulate blood sugar, and lower the chances of diabetes and heart disease. Examples of grains include whole wheat, oats, brown rice, quinoa, barley, and millet. They provide the body with fiber, vitamin B, and energy to run, play, and grow strong. Popcorn is an example of a whole grain. Opting for whole grains provides sustained energy, which makes them a healthy and delicious choice for meals and snacks daily.

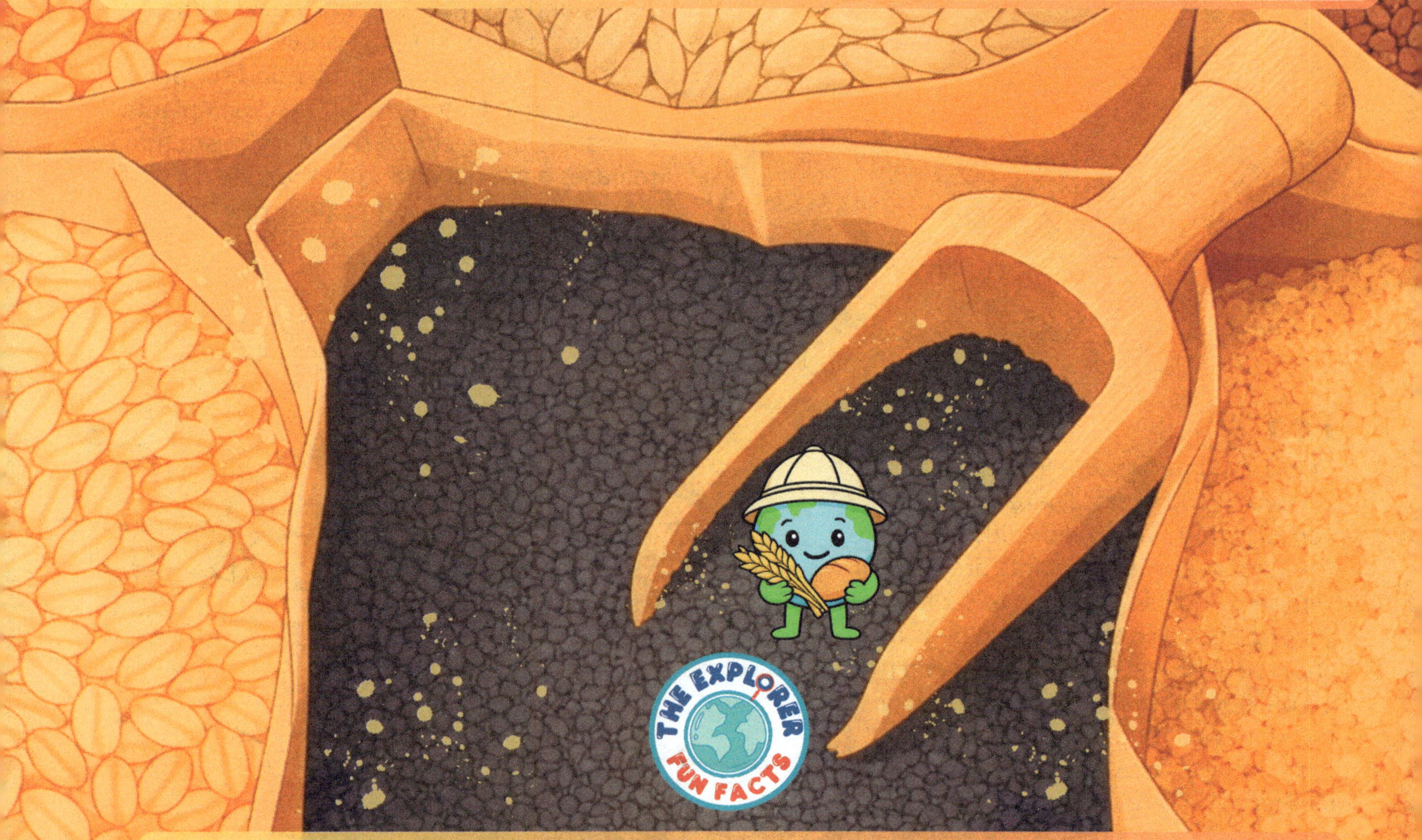

Did you know that the "cereal'" name comes from the Roman goddess Ceres, who was the guardian to safeguard grains.

Whole Wheat

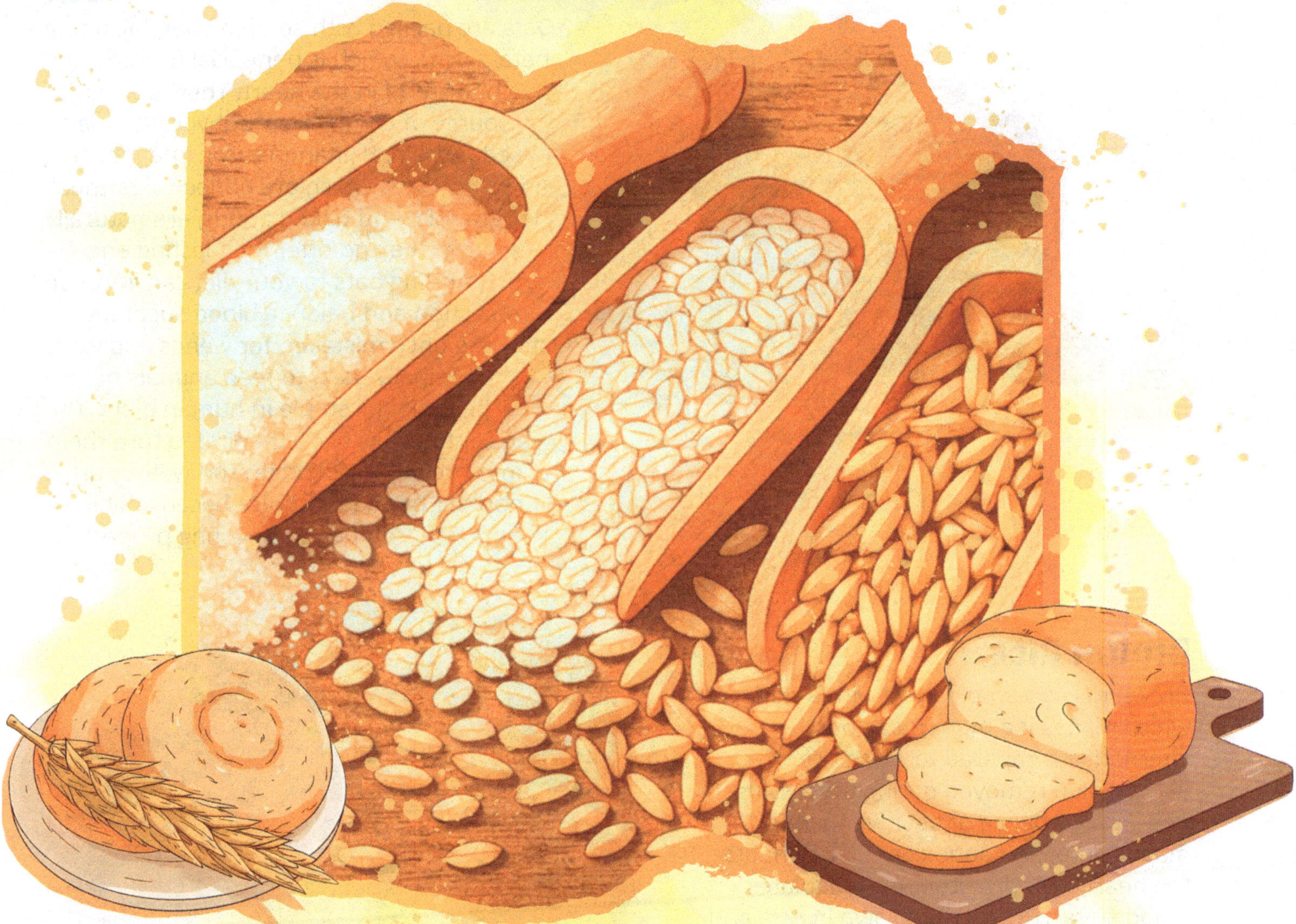

Wheat is a member of the grass family, producing a dry, single-seeded fruit known as a kernel. Whole wheat produces a darker color and firmer texture compared to lighter white wheat, which is softer in texture. Whole wheat provides healthy nutrient content, promoting regularity and a healthy gut microbiome. Bread, pasta, cereal, and crackers made from whole wheat are all examples of complex carbohydrates. Unlike refined grains, whole wheat keeps you feeling full longer and is a smart step toward a long-term balanced diet.

Oat

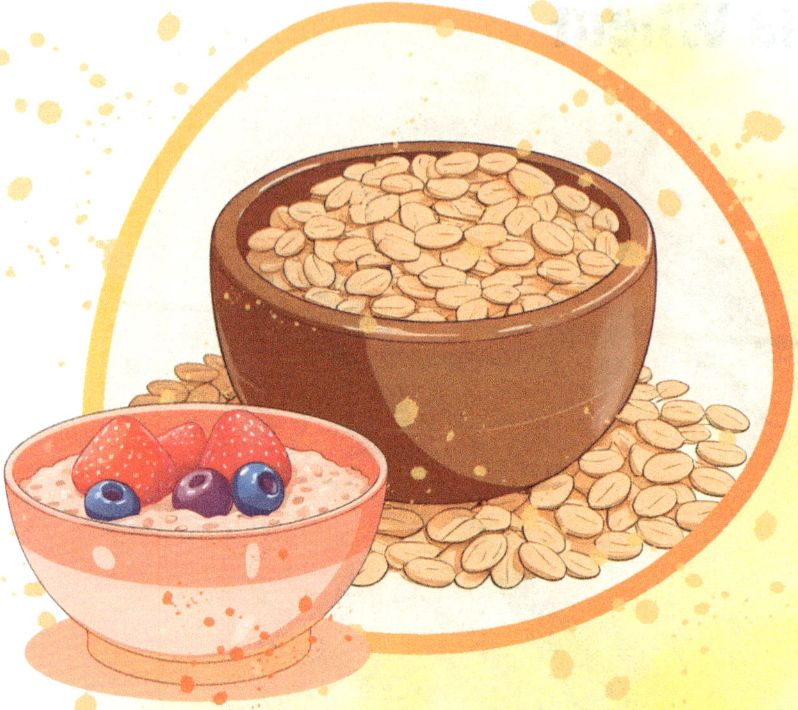

Oats are packed with soluble fiber, including beta-glucan, which is beneficial for reducing cholesterol in the heart. They are a great source of complex carbohydrates, plant-based protein, B vitamins, iron, magnesium, and zinc. Oats, which are added to oatmeal, granola, and baked goods, are naturally gluten-free and offer long-lasting energy. Adding oats to your diet can improve digestion and balance blood sugar levels. Oats were once mistaken for weeds and were initially used to feed animals before becoming a staple in human diets. The ancient Greeks were the first to turn them into breakfast porridge. Today, they are a popular breakfast choice because of their health-boosting properties.

Brown Rice

Brown rice is a whole grain with a skin, which makes it a more nutritious alternative compared to white rice that has the skin removed during processing. It has an abundance of fiber, vitamin B, magnesium, and antioxidants. It benefits the heart, aids digestion, and regulates blood sugar. Brown rice grown in Asia and the Amazon is a healthy swap for your diet, serving as a great source of complex carbohydrates that provide long-lasting energy until your next meal. Brown rice, in contrast to white rice, requires a longer cooking time because of its bran and germ layers, but it is also less processed and more nutritious.

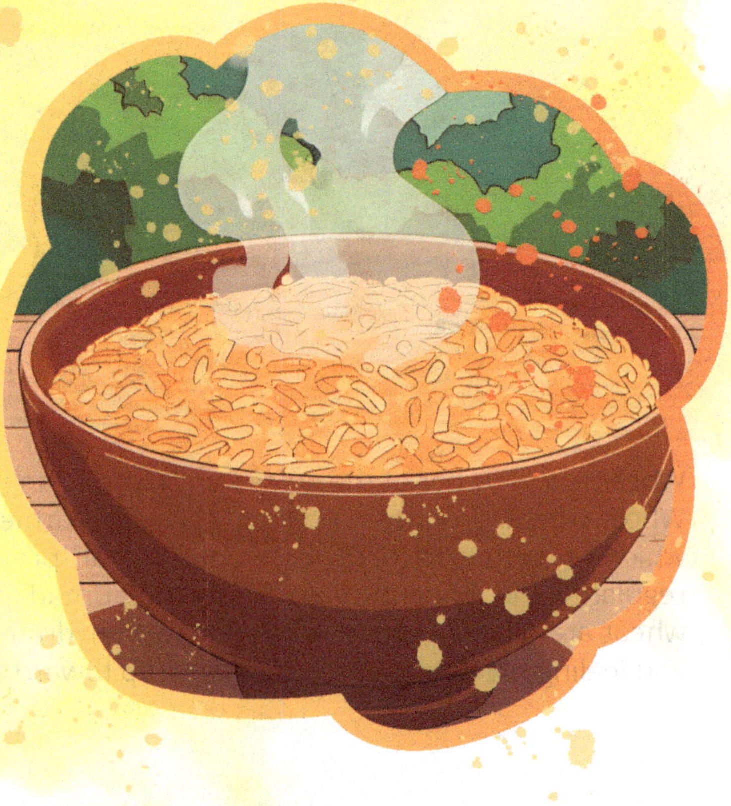

Quinoa

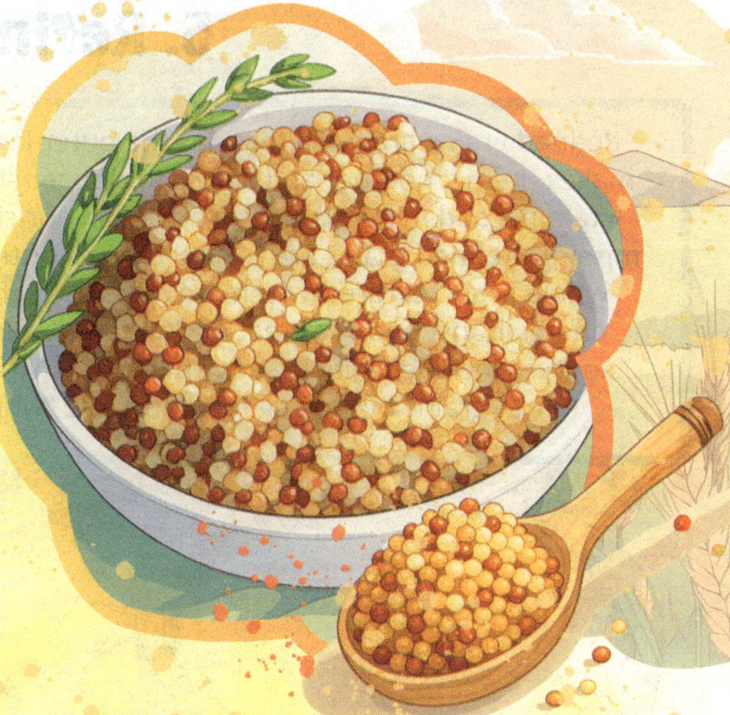

These grains are native to the Andean region of South America and were sacred to the Incas thousands of years ago. Quinoa is a superseed packed with nutrients and is a complete protein containing all nine vital amino acids. Similar to rice, it is easy to prepare by washing and cooking, and is an excellent choice for people with gluten intolerance. Because of its fiber, iron, magnesium, and antioxidant content, quinoa contributes to a healthy heart, digestion, and muscle function. Due to its high nutrient value, NASA has identified quinoa as a suitable crop for space missions. Adding quinoa to your diet boosts plant-based protein intake and supports balanced eating habits for all ages.

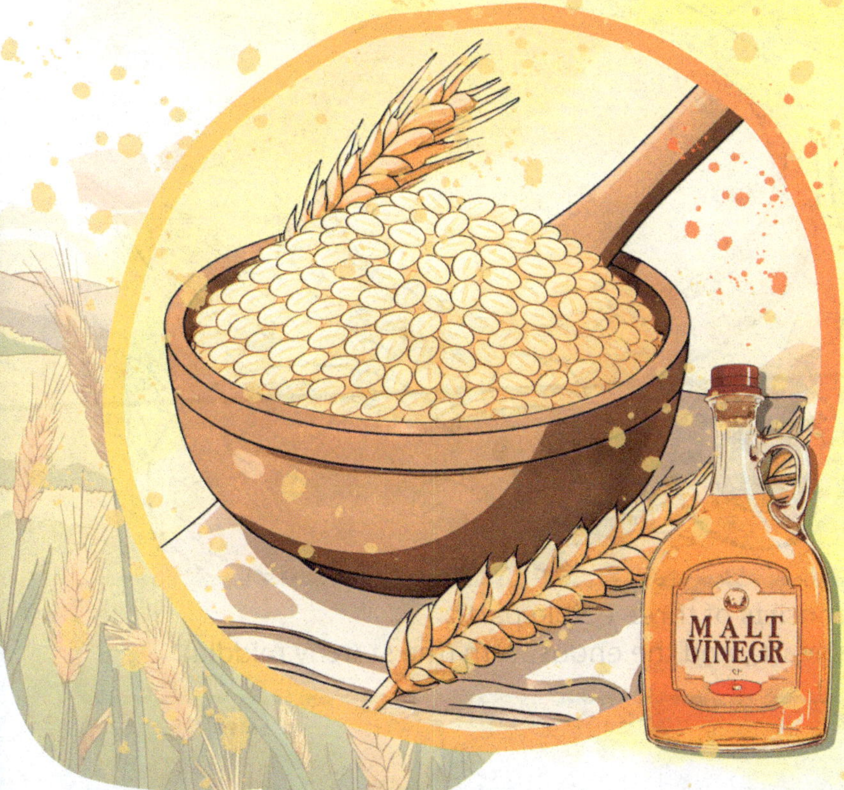

Barley

Barley is a tall grass that was among the earliest grains cultivated by humans. The ancient Romans fed grain to gladiators, and it was also used as a form of currency in ancient Mesopotamia. Barley is a source of soluble fiber, vitamin B, iron, magnesium, phosphorus, and selenium, which help lower cholesterol, stabilize blood sugar, support a healthy heart, aid digestion, and improve energy metabolism. Barley is often added to soups, stews, salads, or eaten as a rice alternative for healthy and balanced nutrition. It is also a key ingredient in the production of malt vinegar.

5. Refined Grains

Refined grains are grain that has the outer layer removed after the milling process. The process makes them smoother and allows for longer storage. While this process removes important fiber, vitamins, and minerals, grains are often enriched to replace essential vitamins and iron that are missing. Refined grains are a good choice for those who prefer a smooth texture, unlike the grainy whole-grain textures, which are difficult to chew. This easily digestible option provides a quick energy boost and is a great option for people with sensitive stomachs. Common refined grain sources include white bread, white pasta, white rice, and flour. You can usually identify refined grains by looking for words like "white flour" or "enriched flour" on the label.

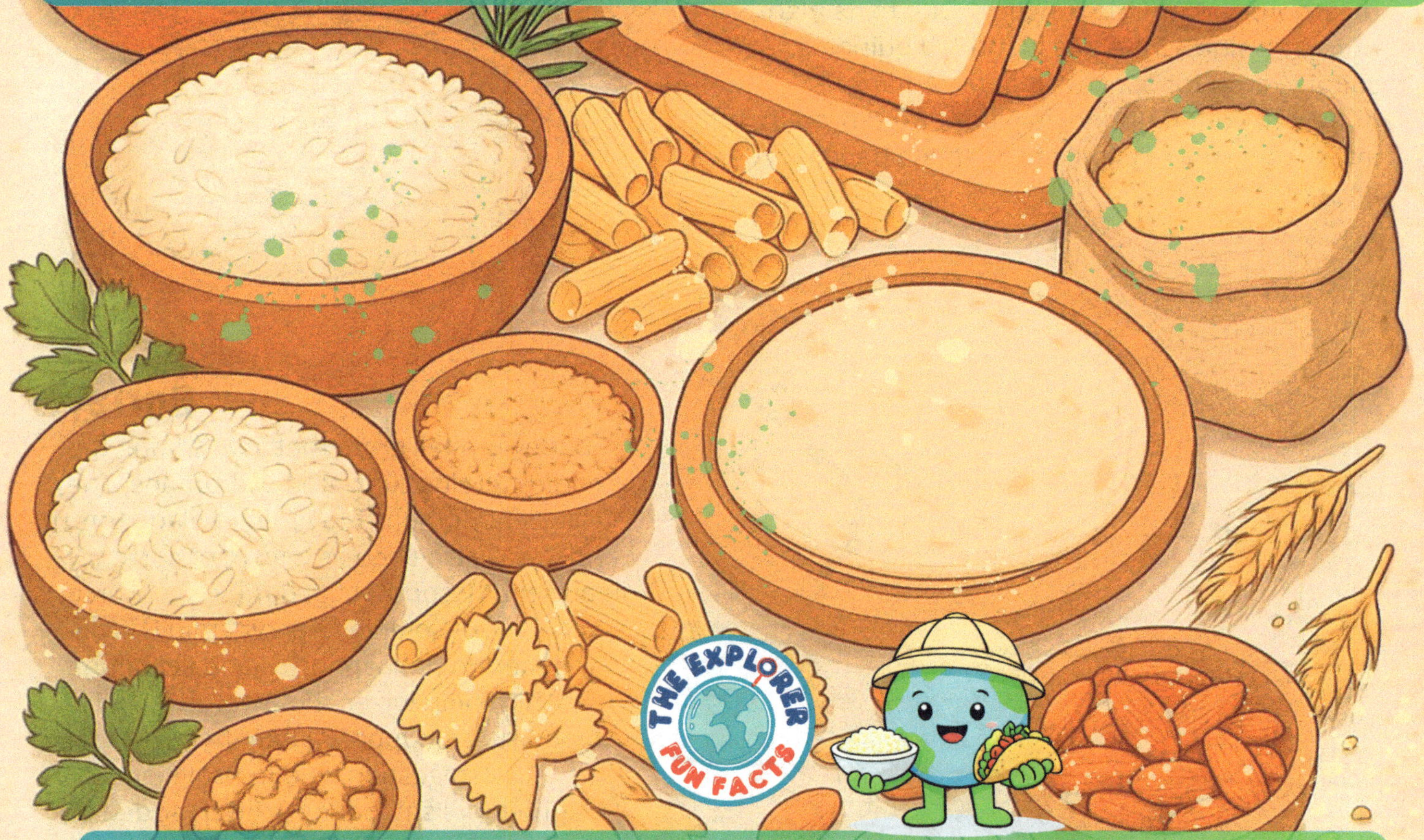

The grain kernel consists of three edible parts:
The bran (outer layer), the germ (the heart), and the endosperm (the starchy middle).

Pasta

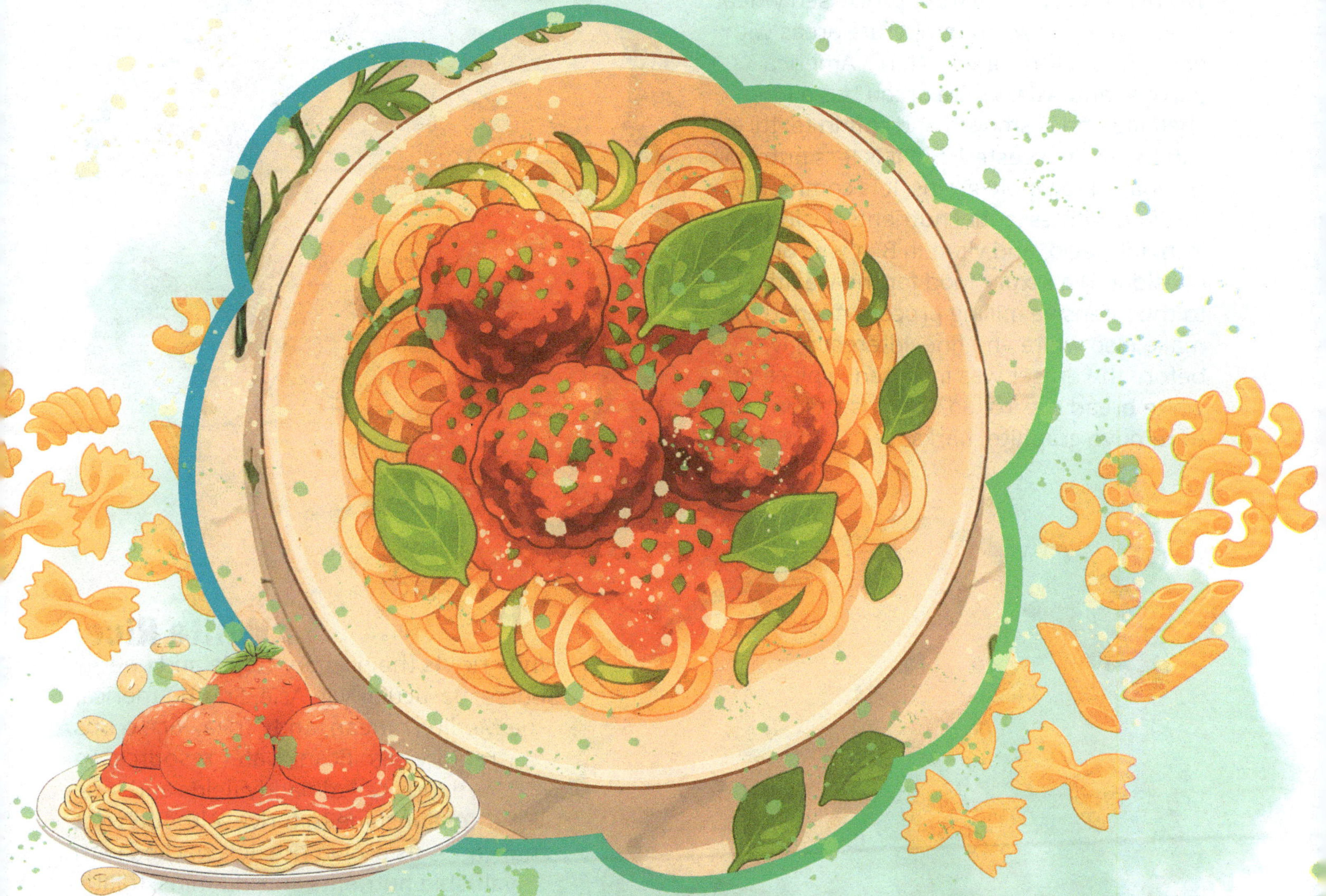

Pasta is made from a type of wheat called durum, which grows in sunny regions across the Mediterranean, the American Midwest, and parts of Canada. While more than 600 types of pasta are available worldwide, their origins trace back to Italy, where different varieties evolved to suit local ingredients and traditions. Pasta is made from simple ingredients, including flour, water, and eggs, and pairs easily with sauces, vegetables, proteins, or olive oil. It is a great source of carbohydrates, vitamin B, and iron, all of which give us energy and keep us feeling full longer. Compared to white bread, pasta has a lower glycemic index and provides more steady energy without dramatic blood sugar spikes.

White Bread

White bread is made from processed wheat flour that is grown in temperate areas with enough rain throughout North America, Europe, and Asia. White bread has a long shelf life and is smooth and soft in texture, can be easily digested, but it is less nutritious compared to whole grains. It is commonly fortified with essential nutrients, including iron, folic acid, and vitamin B. It was once considered a luxury food for the wealthy due to the intensive milling process needed to make it so white and fine. Interestingly, before the eraser was invented, a piece of white bread was rolled up to use as an eraser to remove graphite marks.

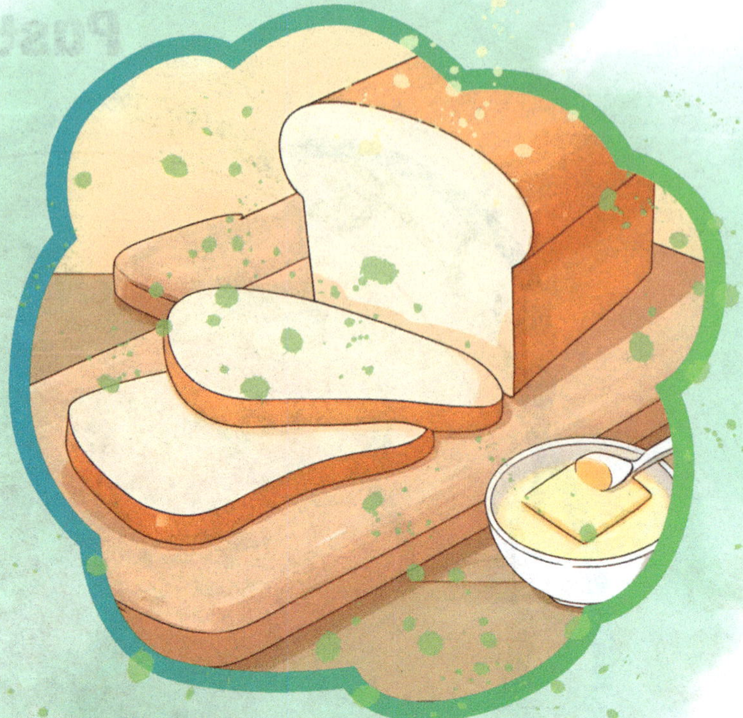

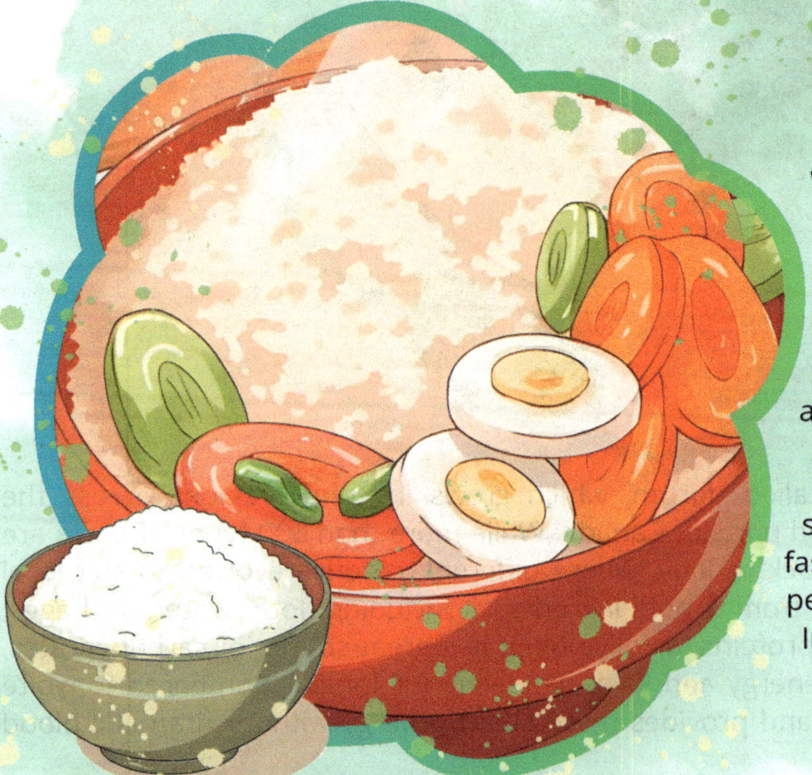

White Rice

White rice is the primary staple and energy source, particularly in Asia, South America, the Mediterranean, and Africa. Rice crops require significant water resources in wetlands called paddy fields and long periods of sunshine to thrive. Although not as nutritious as brown rice, it is packed with valuable nutrients and vitamins, folate, niacin, and iron. White rice can be boiled, steamed, or fried. It is rich in carbs, offering fast and readily absorbed energy suitable for people who are busy or need energy quickly. In Asian cultures, rice represents prosperity and abundance and is often used to add festivity to festivals and weddings.

Flour Tortilla

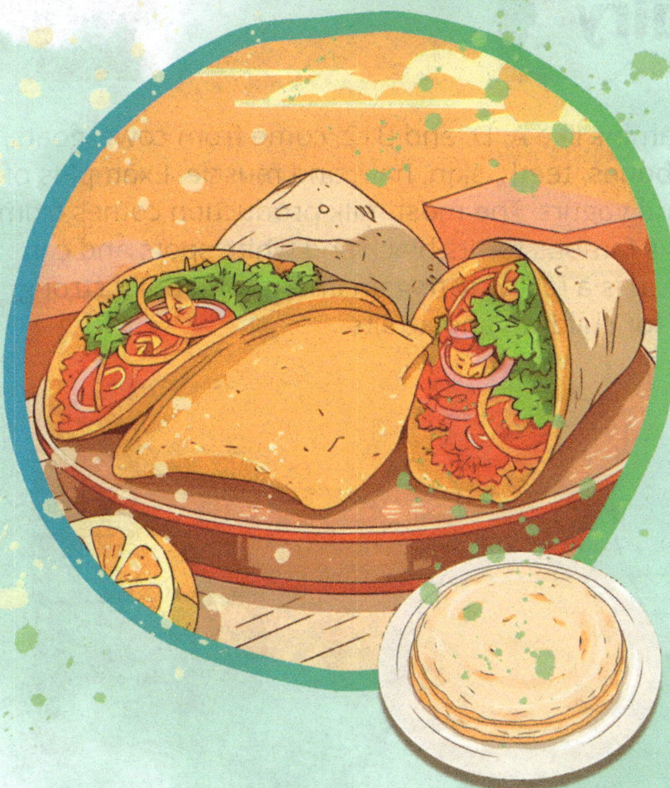

Flour tortillas made from refined wheat flour, water, salt, and fat are soft, flexible, and perfect for holding all kinds of delicious fillings such as vegetables, meats, cheese, and beans for wraps, tacos, quesadillas, and burritos. Nutritionally, tortillas are a quick-energy food rich in carbohydrates, enriched with iron and vitamin B, which are super important for growing kids. Flour tortillas are quick to prepare, easy to store, and fit into many dishes from breakfasts, lunches, and dinners, making them a favorite among kids. They are easier to digest than some bread, perfect for those with digestive issues. The Spanish word “torta,” which translates to “little cake,” is where the word “tortilla” comes from. In space, astronauts prefer tortillas over bread because they don't create floating crumbs that could damage equipment or incidentally get inhaled.

Couscous

Couscous isn’t a grain but actually a type of pasta made from semolina wheat that is a staple in North Africa and Mediterranean cuisine. It is cultivated in sunny and semi-arid climates in the Maghreb region. This light and fluffy granulated grain is an excellent source of vitamin B, fiber, protein, and carbohydrates for quick energy, and antioxidants from selenium. It is simple to cook by adding vegetables, herbs, meats, or adding to a stew or salad, making it an easy, satisfying, and balanced dish for busy people who want something nutritious without the fuss.

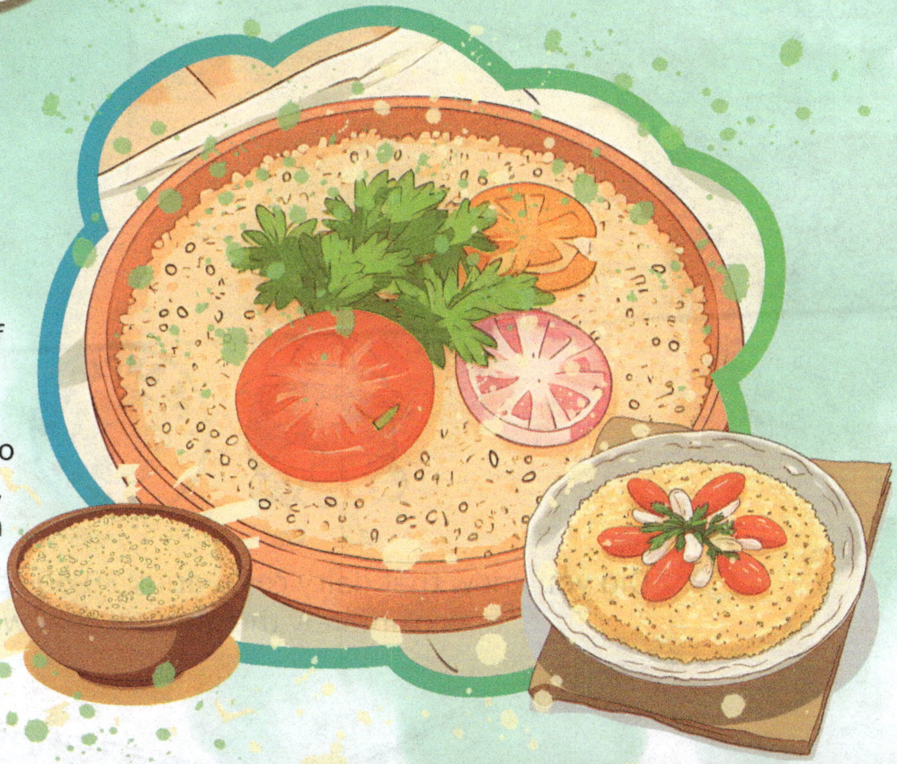

6. Dairy

Dairy products are rich in calcium, protein, and vitamins like A, D, and B12, come from cows, goats, and sheep. These nutrients contribute to healthy bones, teeth, skin, hair, and muscle. Examples of dairy products include ice cream, butter, cheese, and yogurt. The most milk production comes from the popular dairy breed, the Holstein cow, which is famous for its black and white spots and can give several gallons of milk daily. Dairy consumption is a fast way to gain energy and build strong bones, which is beneficial for children and adults.

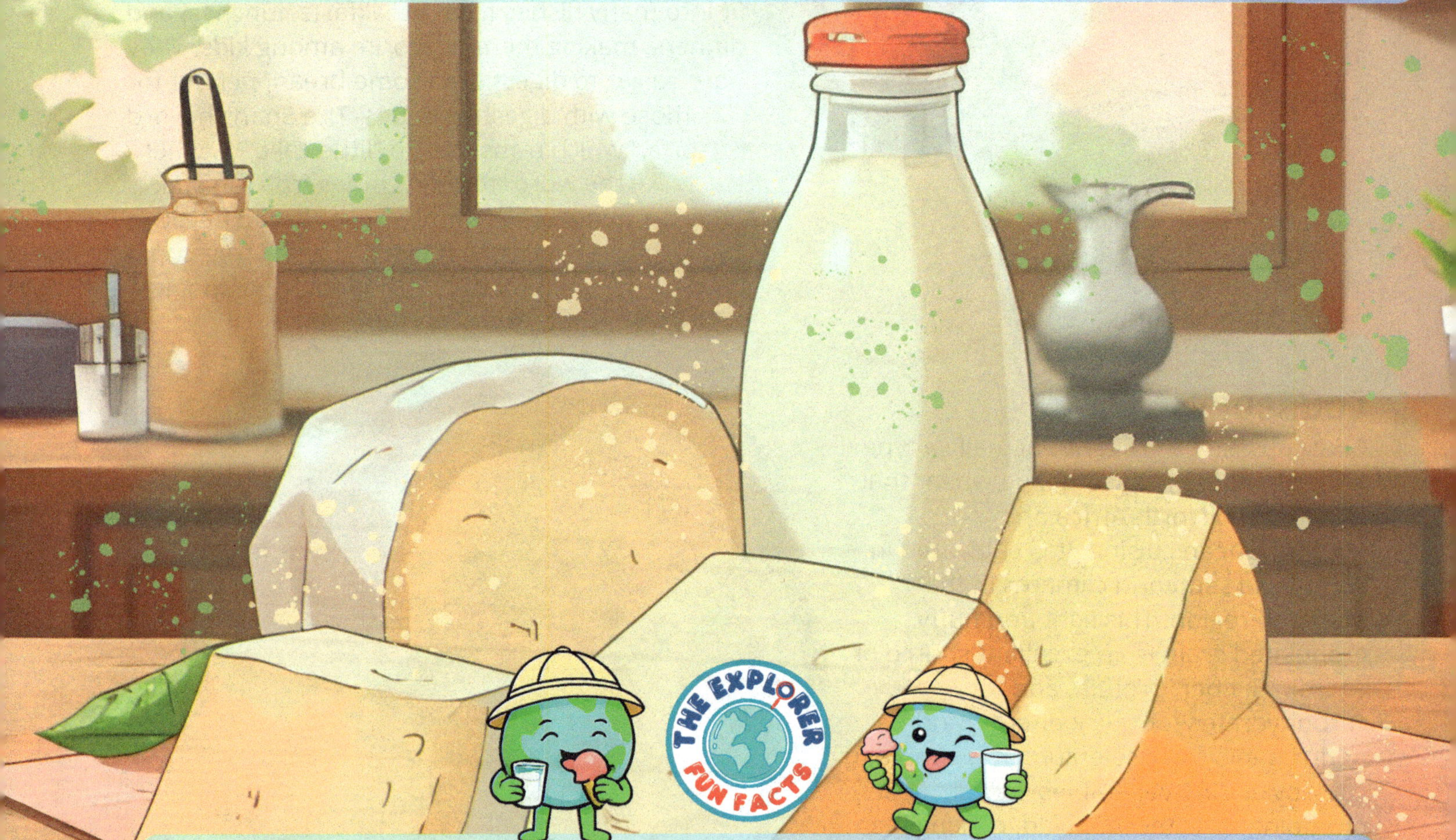

Did you know that dairy cows drink 30-50 gallons of water daily, which is approximately the amount that would fill a bathtub?

Milk

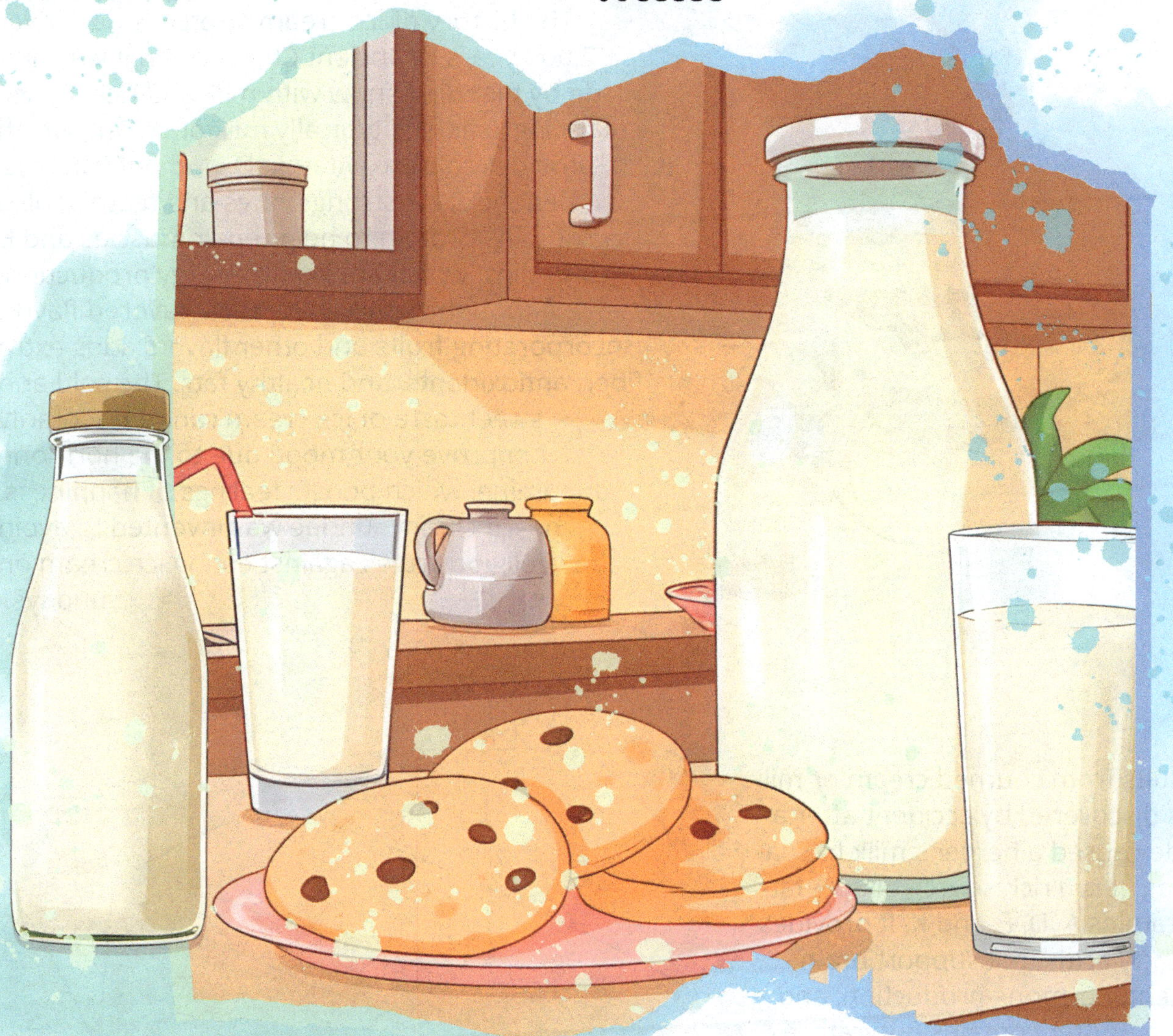

Milk is a source of calcium, protein, vitamin D, and potassium. The calcium found in milk can help protect against bone diseases, such as osteoporosis, as people age. Milk is used to make a variety of foods, including cheese, yogurt, and butter. Besides its nutritional benefits, milk is used to produce biodegradable bioplastics, and the lactic acid it contains serves as a natural moisturizer for the skin. Milk contains over 85% water, appears white because its fat and protein molecules reflect and scatter light, but it's actually slightly bluish in its natural state. Milk can soothe your mouth after a spicy meal, thanks to the casein protein, which cleanses your taste buds.

Ice Cream

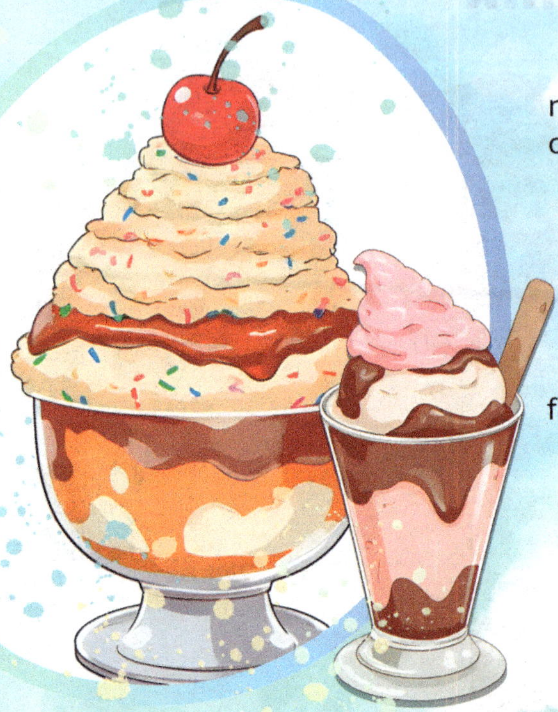

The history of ice cream stretches back over 2,000 years to ancient China, when it was first made by blending snow with milk and rice. An ice cream ingredient is typically milk or cream, which provides calcium, vitamin D, and phosphorus, beneficial for strong bones and teeth. It also contains protein to help repair muscles and B vitamins, which are key to energy production. Although vanilla is the most favored flavor, incorporating fruits and other flavors adds extra fiber, antioxidants, and healthy fats. The cold and sweet taste of ice cream can momentarily improve your mood due to the hormone dopamine, which boosts feelings of happiness. The ice cream sundae was invented to avoid religious rules against eating ice cream on Sundays.

Butter

Butter results from churned cream or milk, and it was discovered by accident after a bumpy ride caused a herder's milk to shake within a bag. It is a rich source of 80% fat-soluble vitamins A, D, E, and K. It provides essential fatty acids that support brain development, hormone production, and healthy skin. Butter contains butyrate, a short-chain fatty acid that promotes gut health and reduces inflammation. Butter improves the flavor of meals and provides energy to growing children. The ancient Romans used butter as a food, medicine, and skin cream. Including small amounts in a balanced diet can support nutrition and taste.

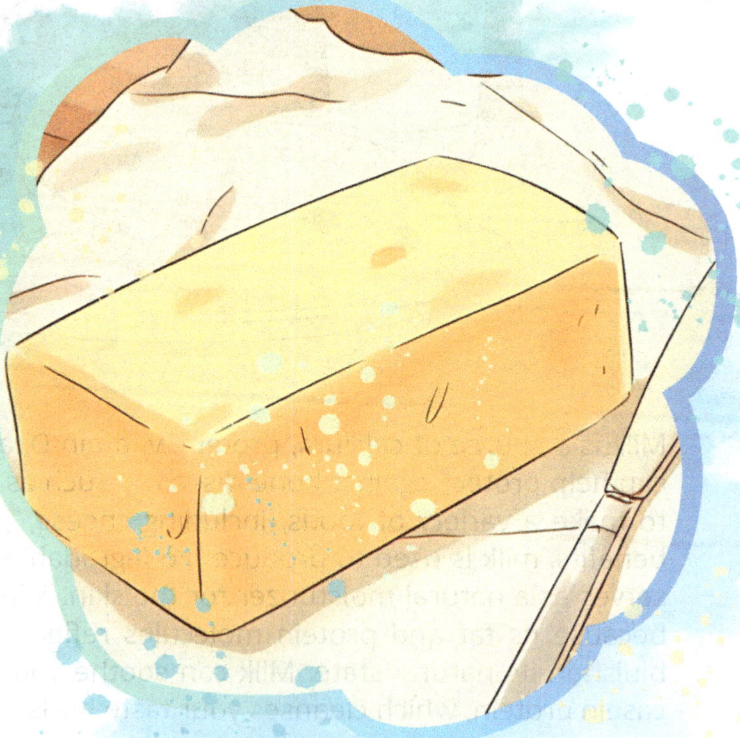

Cheese

Cheese is made from cow, goat, or sheep's milk that was created by accident over 4,000 years ago when people stored milk in animal stomachs. There are over 2000 different varieties of cheese known around the world. Cheese is rich in calcium, protein, vitamin B12, zinc, and phosphorus, which are essential for strong bones and healthy teeth, support muscle growth, energy production, and nerve function. Cheese contains healthy fats that contribute to satiety and flavor in meals. Some cheeses offer probiotics that aid digestion and a healthy gut. Eating in moderation in your diet can enhance nutrient intake, especially for growing children and older adults needing bone support. The stretchy proteins in cheese are responsible for the "squeak" that you hear when you eat it.

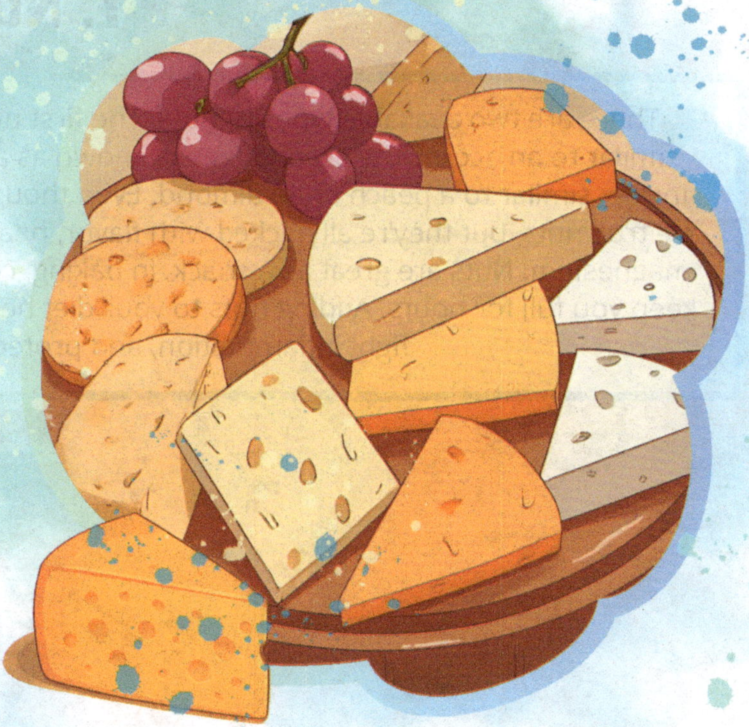

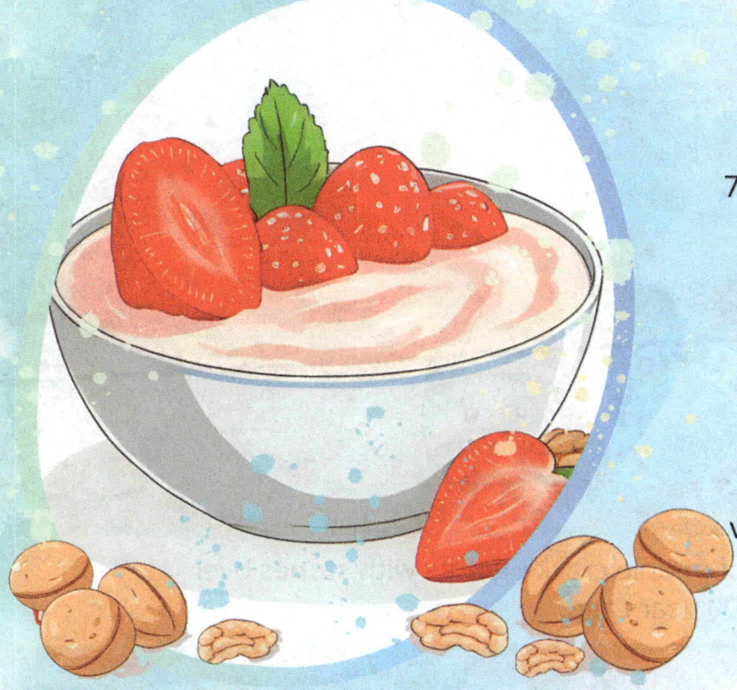

Yogurt

Yogurt is made from cow, goat, or plant-based milk, such as almond or soy. Yogurt is an ancient food, discovered by accident around 7,000 B.C. when Nomadic people carried milk in animal-skin pouches, and the natural bacteria and warm temperatures turned it into yogurt. The word yogurt comes from the Turkish word “yoğ”, which means “to condense” or “to thicken”. The distinctive thickness and tart flavor of yogurt result from fermenting heated milk with beneficial bacteria like Lactobacillus and Bifidobacterium. It is rich in calcium, vitamin B12, protein, riboflavin, potassium, and probiotics that support gut health, a healthy immune system, strengthen bones, boost immunity, and help maintain a healthy weight when added to a balanced diet.

7. Nuts

There are two available types of nuts. The first nut is a dry, single seed fruit with a hard shell, similar to an acorn. The second type is known as a drupe with a soft outer part and a hard seed inside, similar to a peach or an almond. Even though we call many of them "nuts," not all of them are true nuts, but they're all packed with flavor, healthy nutrients, fats, protein, fiber, vitamins, and magnesium. Nuts are great as a snack, in baking, cooking, salads, or blended into smoothies, and keep you full for hours. Adding nuts to your diet helps keep your heart, brain, and muscles strong, fight inflammation, and protect your cells from damage.

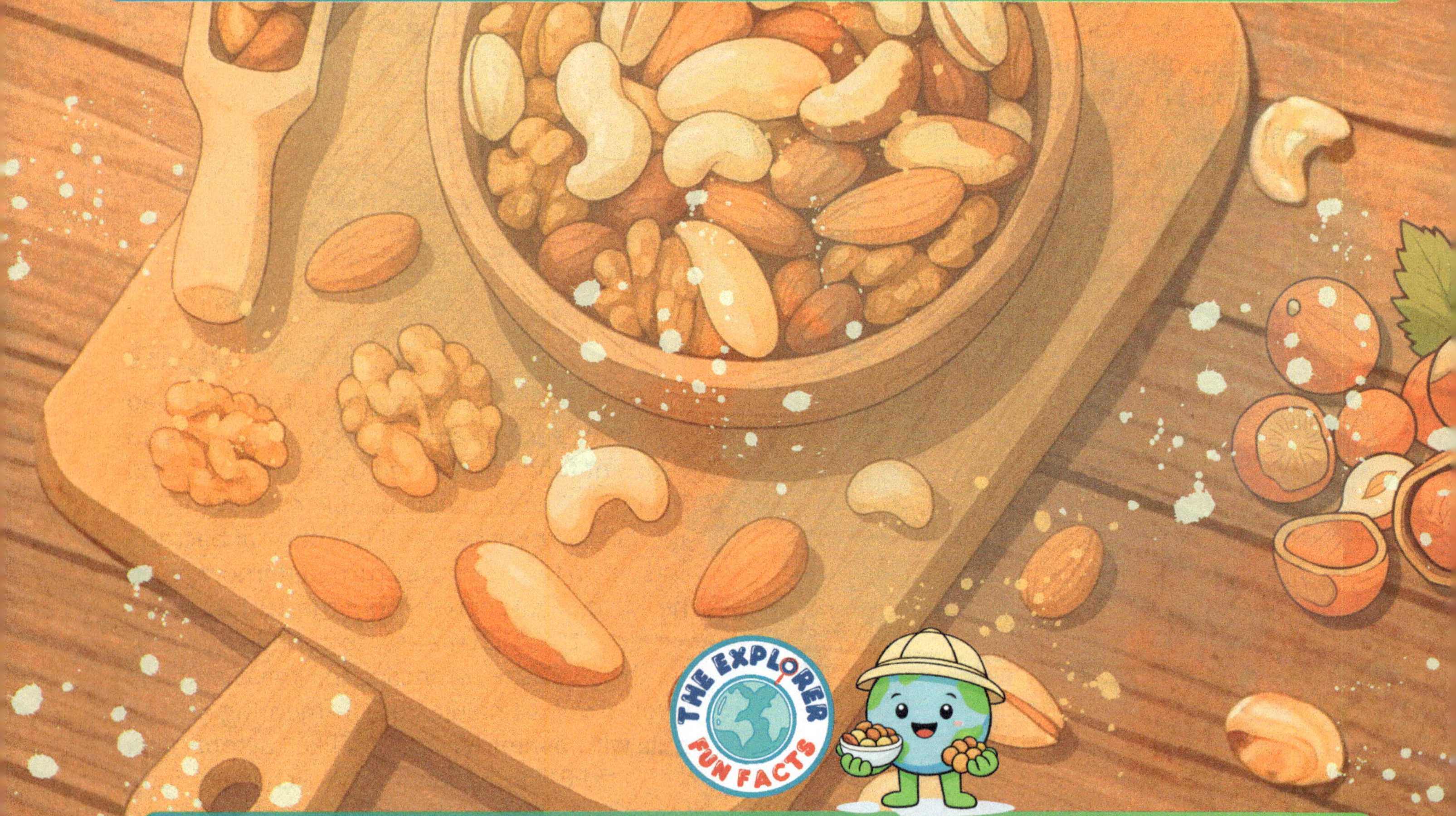

THE EXPLORER FUN FACTS

Archaeologists found evidence of people cracking nuts with stones over 780,000 years ago.

Almond

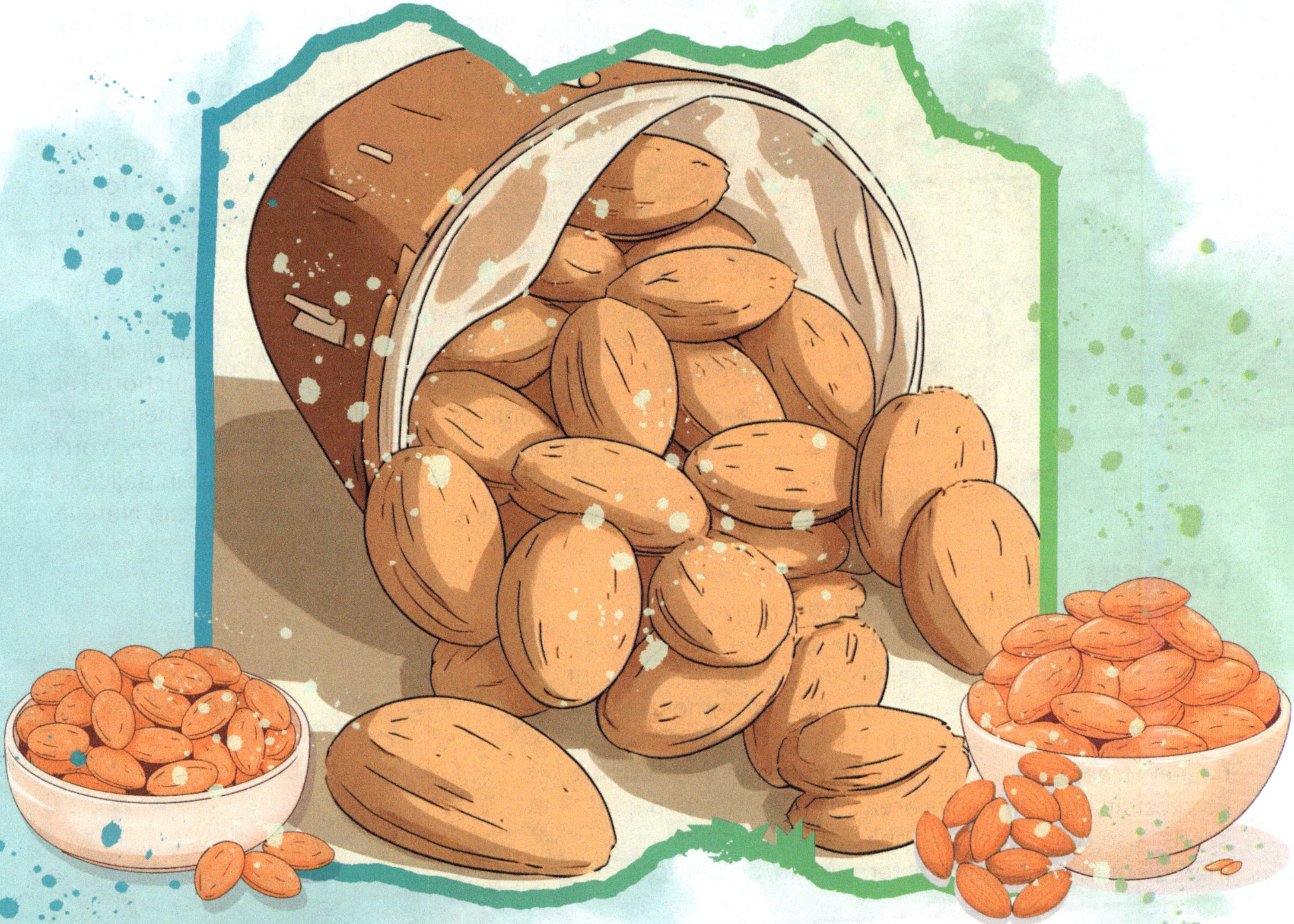

Almonds are not actually nuts but a fruit related to peaches that grows in Mediterranean climates like California and Spain. These ancient superfoods are an excellent source of healthy fats, protein, fiber, vitamin E, magnesium, and antioxidants. Almonds contain nutrients that support heart health, brain function, blood sugar control, and promote satiety, making them ideal for daily snacks. You can eat them raw, roasted, as almond butter, or milk. Almonds add flavor, crunch, and essential nutrients to support overall well-being and diet. In many cultures, almonds are associated with good luck and prosperity and are often given as gifts on special occasions.

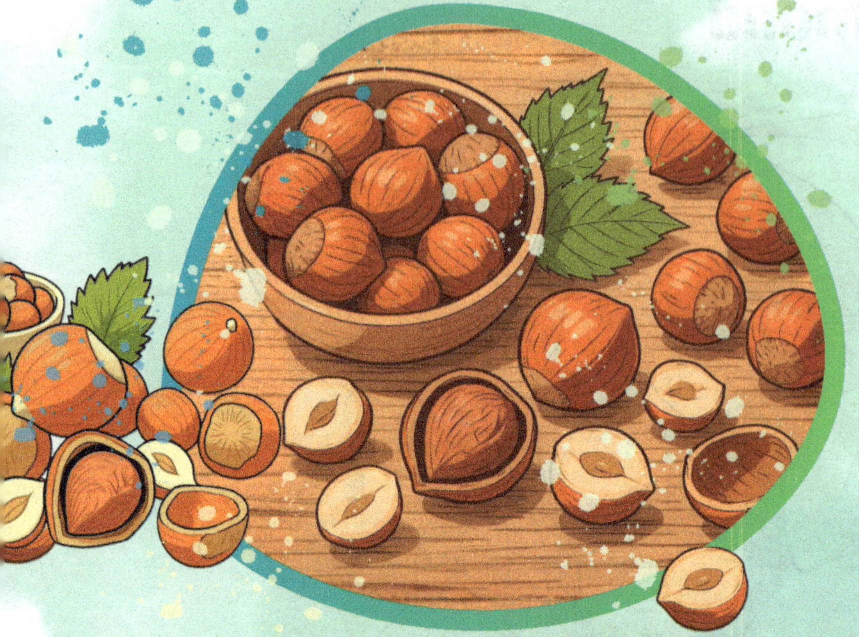

Hazelnut

Hazelnuts grow widely in regions like Turkey, Italy, and Oregon in the US. These little nuts are packed with health benefits. They offer monounsaturated fats, vitamin E, and essential minerals like calcium, manganese, and copper. Hazelnuts are beneficial for the heart by helping lower bad cholesterol and having a high antioxidant count to fight off inflammation. Hazelnuts have the highest concentration of folate of any tree nut. Folate is important, especially for red blood cell production and proper brain function. The antioxidants in hazelnuts may even help make your skin strong against the sun's rays. You'll often find them as a key ingredient in delicious things, like the famous spread, Nutella.

Cashew

Cashews are nutrient-dense tree nuts native to northeastern Brazil that were brought to other continents by Portuguese sailors in the 1560s. This plant thrives in sandy coastal and tropical environments such as in India, Vietnam, and certain regions of Africa. Cashew trees can help prevent soil erosion and support biodiversity in their native areas. These kidney-shaped seeds, also called cashew apples, are a popular ingredient in the Middle Eastern, Asian, and African cuisines.

Cashew is rich in healthy monounsaturated fats, protein, magnesium, zinc, and copper to support heart health, bone strength, brain function, and immunity. It provides essential amino acids and antioxidants to combat inflammation. It offers complete protein, which is often lacking in vegetarian meals. Just like almonds, cashews aren't actual nuts, but they are seeds with toxic oil shells that require careful processing before consumption to prevent skin rashes.

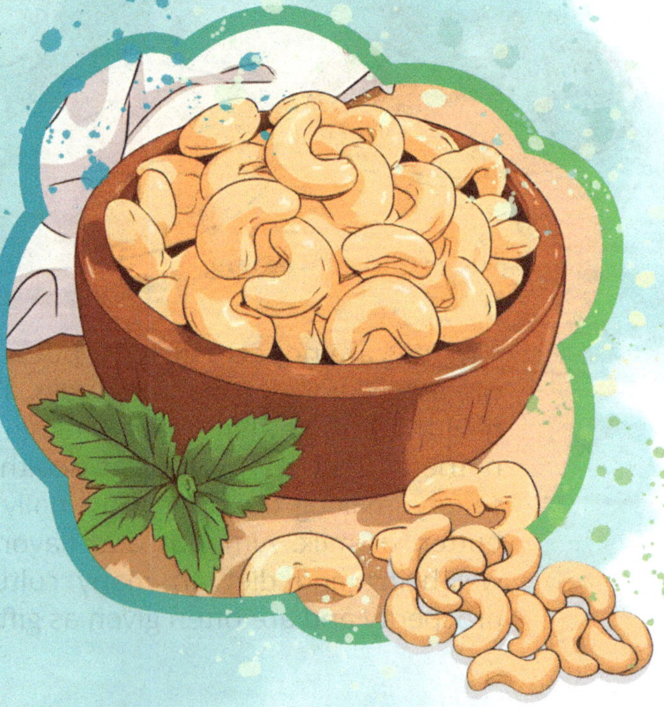

Walnut

Scientists think humans consumed this ancient food many millennia ago in the early Neolithic period. Walnut has a distinctive flavor, texture, and nutritional benefits, making it a popular baking and savory cooking ingredient. It flourishes in temperate environments with good drainage and naturally grows from the Balkans to the Himalayas. Nowadays, it is widely cultivated in California, China, Iran, and Turkey. Walnut is rich in omega-3 fatty acids, making them a popular plant-based fish omega substitution for vegans. They also provide fiber, vitamin E, magnesium, and antioxidants, which support heart health, brain function, and reduce inflammation. As a renewable resource, walnut shells are also used in eco-friendly products. Walnut's shape resembles the human brain. Including them in your diet naturally boosts memory and cognitive function.

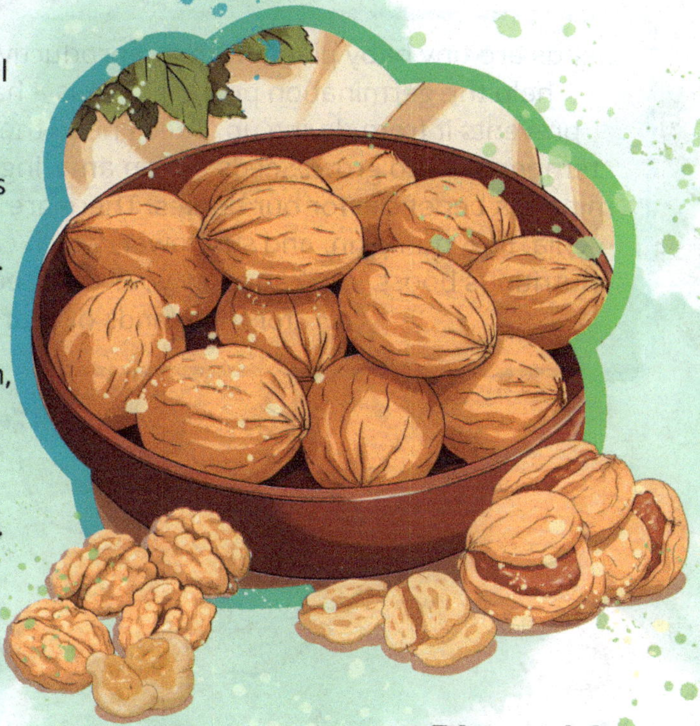

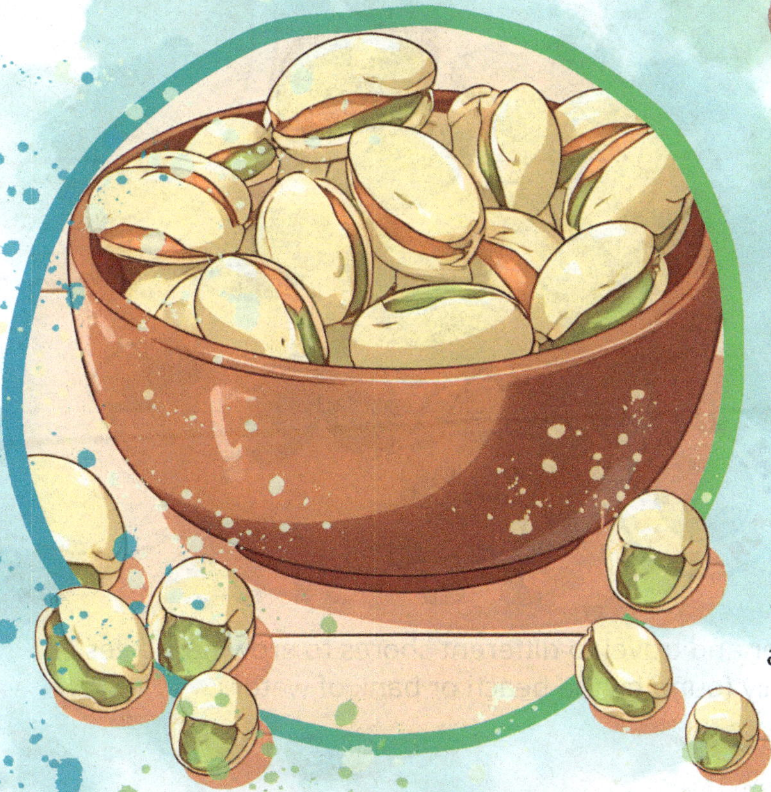

Pistachio

Pistachios grow in dry climates with hot summers and cool winters and are native to arid regions in Central Asia, the Middle East, and the Mediterranean. The trees can live for a very long time, sometimes up to 300 years. Frequently used in Middle Eastern, Mediterranean, Italian, and Indian cooking, they are ideal for various dishes, including desserts, pastries, and savory meals. Pistachios are rich in protein, healthy fats, fiber, potassium, and vitamin B6, which are beneficial for regulating blood sugar levels. These are packed with antioxidants like lutein and zeaxanthin, which support good vision. In China, they are called "happy nuts" due to their shells opening into a shape that resembles a smile.

8. Seeds

Seeds are tiny baby plants with a reproductive unit containing a small embryo and a food source to help the germination process. It has a hard shell or coat that acts as a protective layer and prevents it from drying up. Seeds need the right amount of soil, water, oxygen, and the correct temperature to grow. Seeds are an amazing source of nutrients, protein, fats, fiber, vitamins, and minerals beneficial for our bodies. There are many delicious and healthy seeds to snack on, such as chia, flax, pumpkin, and sunflower, which can be sprinkled on yogurt, salads, or smoothies for a nutritious boost. You can grow your own seed and watch it grow. Certain seeds can stay dormant for thousands of years before sprouting new plants.

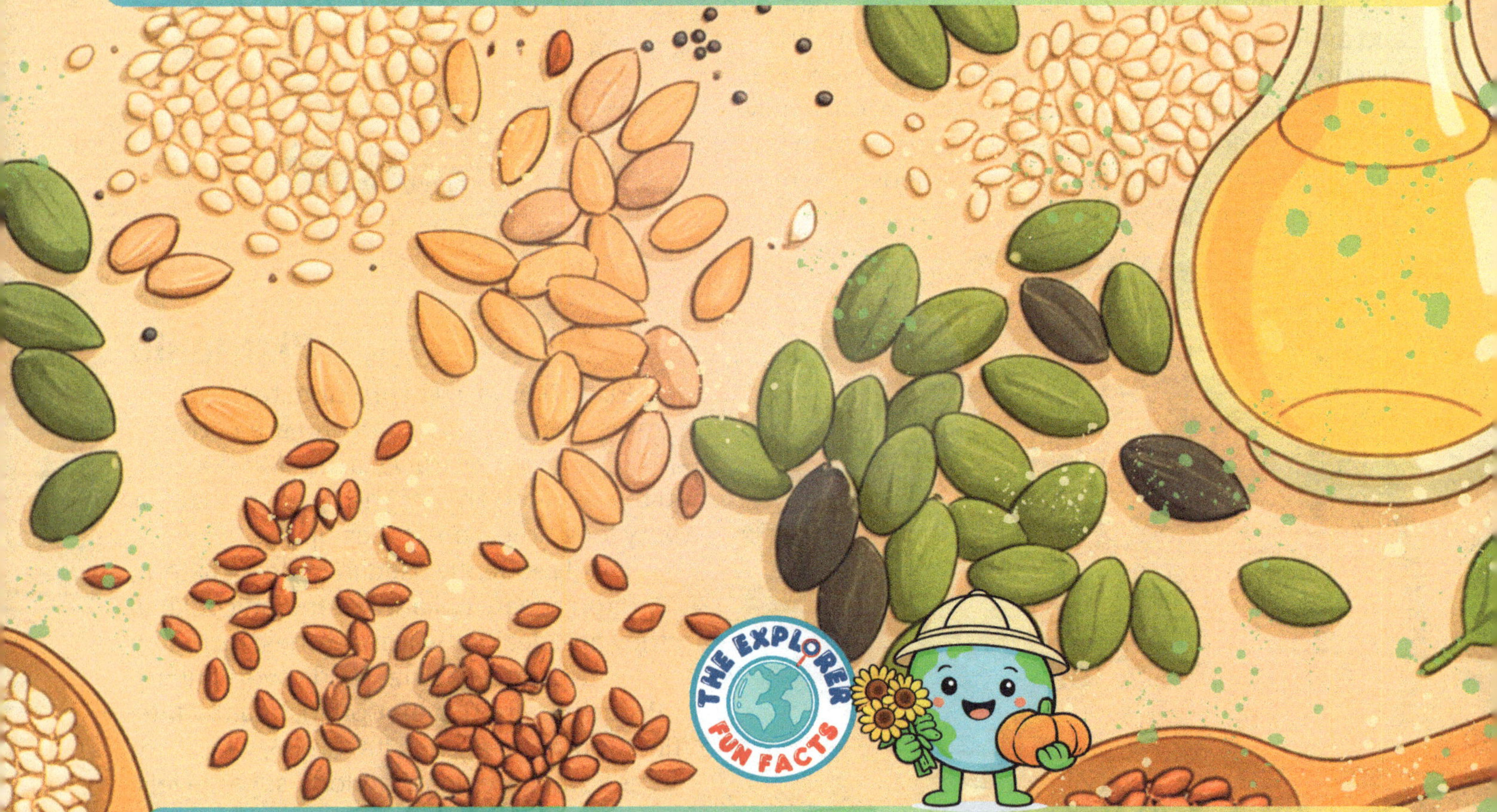

A coconut is a seed that can float in water and travel to different shores to grow new trees. No wonder they are commonly found by the beach or bank of water.

Chia Seed

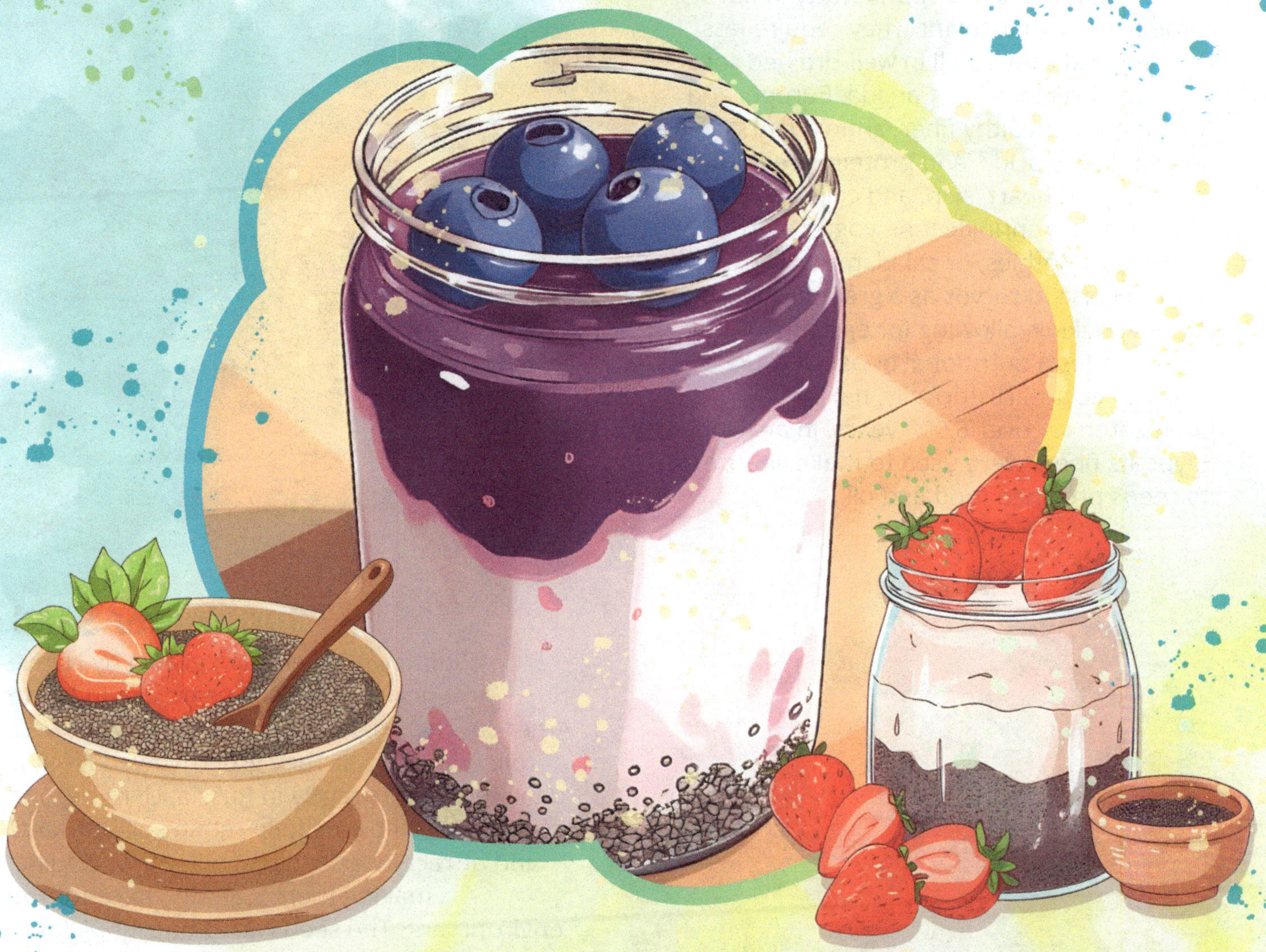

Chia seeds are tiny but packed with powerful benefits. They come from a flowering plant native to Central and South America. Chia seeds thrive in dry, sunny desert climates and are harvested from tall, green stalks. It is full of omega-3 fats that help brain development, calcium for strong bones, fiber for digestion, protein for growth, and antioxidants to protect cells from damage. When soaked in water, chia seeds puff up into a gel, making them fun to eat and helpful for hydration. A spoonful added to yogurt, smoothies, or oatmeal keeps you feeling full longer. The ancient Aztec warriors ate chia seeds to replenish their energy for a whole day. It is also great as an egg replacement on a plant-based diet.

Flaxseed

Flaxseeds, which are tiny and nutty in flavor, come from the flax plant. They require less fertilizer and thrive well in well-drained soils and cooler regions like Canada, Europe, and Asia. It offers healthy fiber, antioxidants, omega-3 fatty acids, and protein, great for keeping your heart, skin, and cells healthy. You can easily sprinkle it on yogurt, cereal, granola, smoothies, or salad, much like chia seeds. Flaxseed serves as a great binding agent in baking, allowing for egg substitutions, and provides a nutritional boost to your favorite recipes. Historically, flaxseeds have been eaten for over 6,000 years. In ancient Egypt, its fibers were used to make linen, and its seeds provided food and oil.

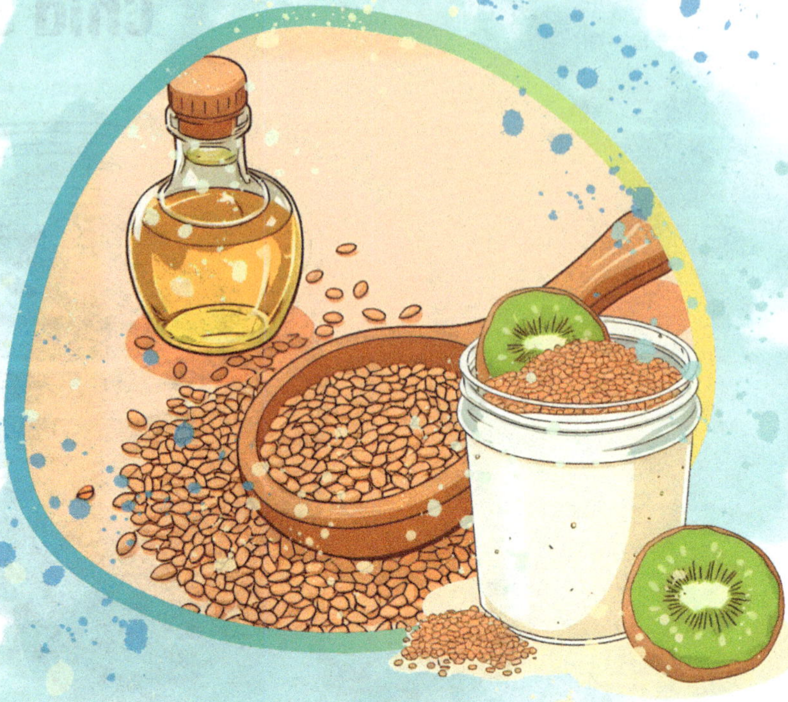

Sunflower Seed

Sunflowers were first grown by Native Americans over 5000 years ago in North America. The bright and vibrant yellow flowers follow the sun as they grow. Nowadays, it is cultivated commercially in Russia, Ukraine, and Argentina. Sunflowers help retain soil nutrients and attract insects, birds, and other wildlife, making them a great choice for the environment. The seeds are a nutritious food, high in vitamin E, healthy fats, protein, and minerals that are important for our muscles and nerves, and can be consumed raw, roasted, or as butter. They contain a nutrient called choline, which is crucial for helping your brain function properly. So, when you're snacking on sunflower seeds, you're not just getting a tasty treat but also giving your brain a little boost.

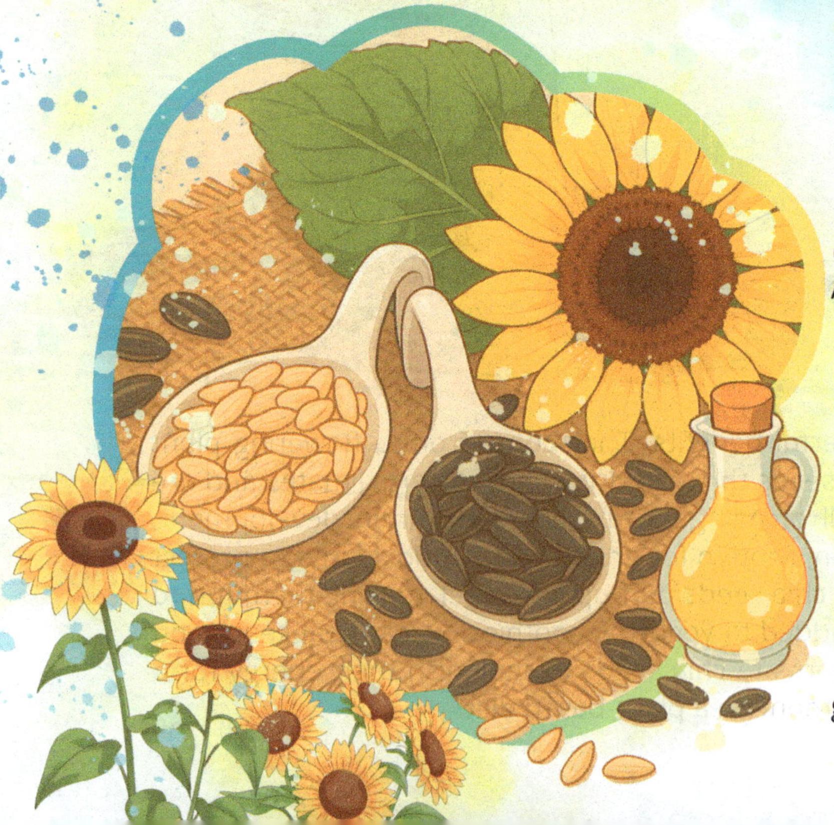

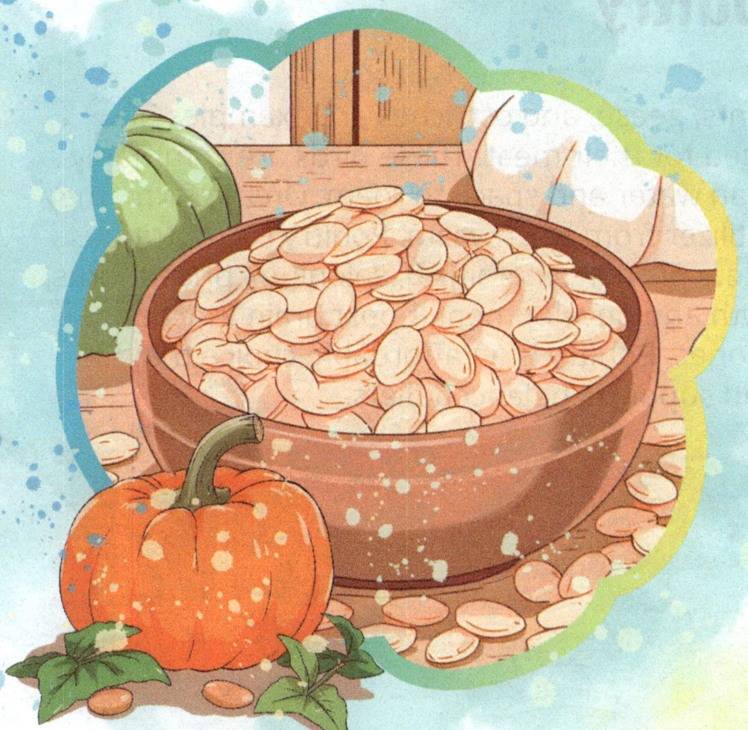

Pumpkin Seed

Pumpkins belong to the squash family and love sunny and warm climates across North and South America. It flourishes in open fields with rich soil. The seeds have been consumed for over 7000 years in Mexico, typically harvested at the end of the pumpkin season. They are called "pepitas" in Spanish and contain protein and healthy fats, making them great for keeping the heart strong and the body energized. It is also a great source of minerals like magnesium, zinc, and iron that most people don't get enough of in their regular diet. They naturally contain an amino acid that helps the body produce serotonin and melatonin. Eating a small amount of these seeds before you go to sleep may improve your sleep, but remember to brush your teeth afterward.

Sesame Seed

Sesame seeds originated in the Indian subcontinent, and are among the oldest crops grown for their oil. The plant's cultivation spread through trade routes to Mesopotamia, Africa, and eventually to East and Southeast Asia. Today, sesame is grown in many tropical and subtropical climates. Its nutty, sweet, and savory flavor makes it ideal for baking, cooking, garnishing, and it is typically used in a variety of Middle Eastern and Asian cuisines. Sesame seeds are packed with healthy fats, protein, fiber, and minerals, which help keep bones strong and regulate blood pressure. Some say the phrase "open sesame" from the tale "Ali Baba and the Forty Thieves" may have originated from the way sesame pods pop open when ripe, spilling out their seeds.

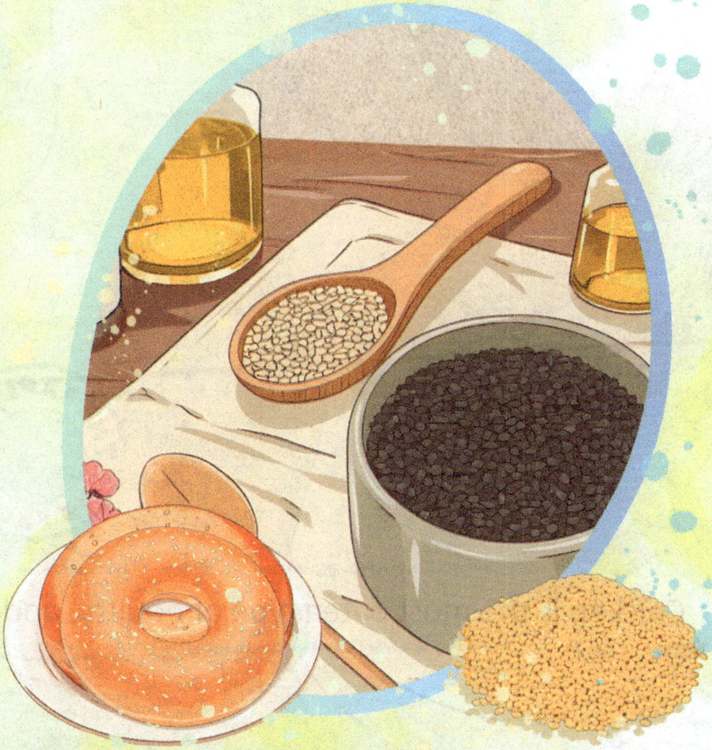

9. Poultry

Chickens, turkeys, hens, ducks, pheasants, geese, and ostriches are examples of domesticated birds that are commonly raised for their meat. These birds are commonly raised on farms or in confined areas with clean water and space to roam. On the farm, they help manage pests and provide natural fertilizer from their waste. Poultry is a nutritious food source of lean meat that offers a complete protein, vitamins B, selenium, phosphorus, zinc, and iron. These nutrients help growth and development, boost brain function, support immune health, and strengthen bones. Poultry is an affordable choice that fits easily into many meals and supports balanced diets.

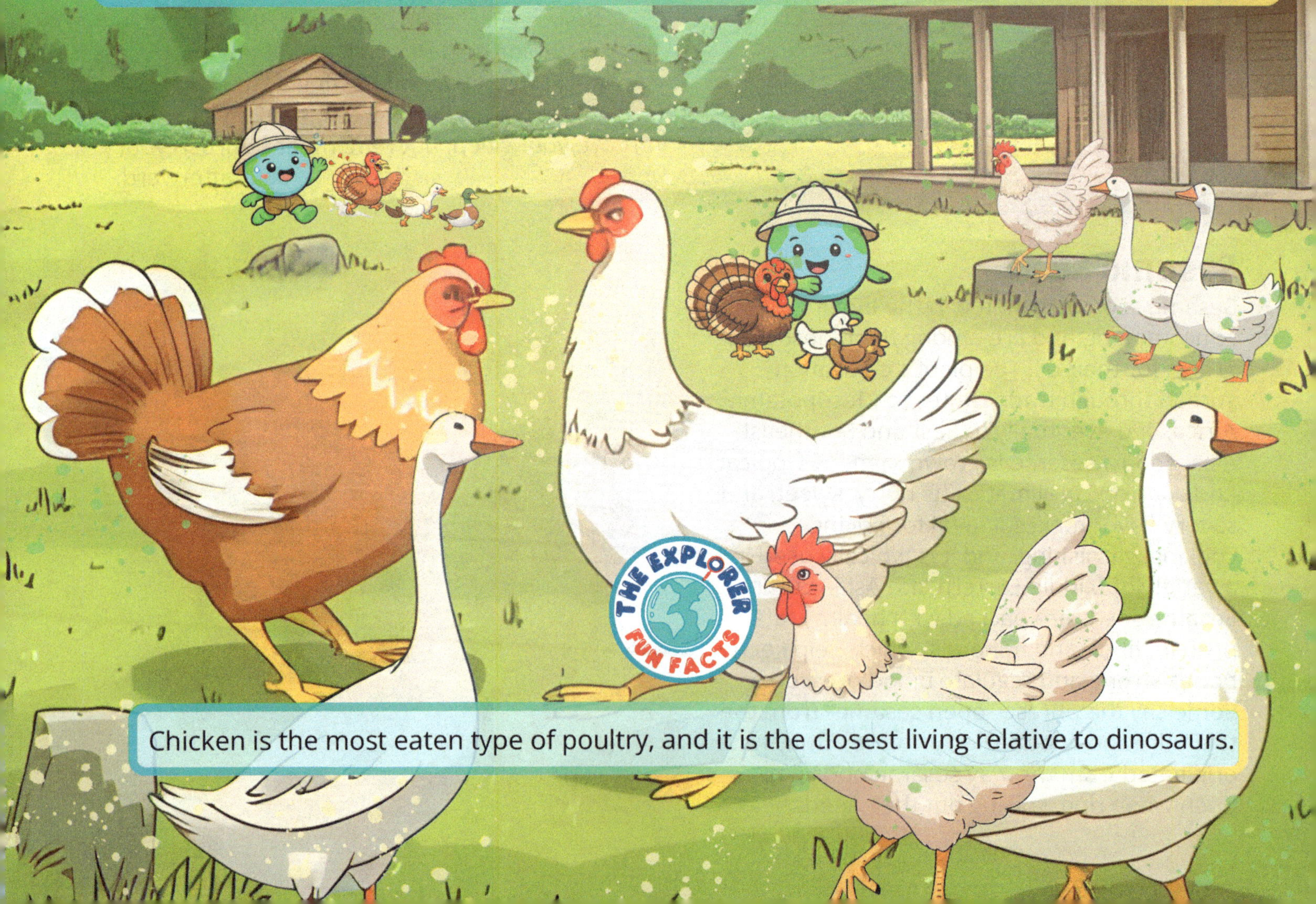

Chicken is the most eaten type of poultry, and it is the closest living relative to dinosaurs.

Chicken

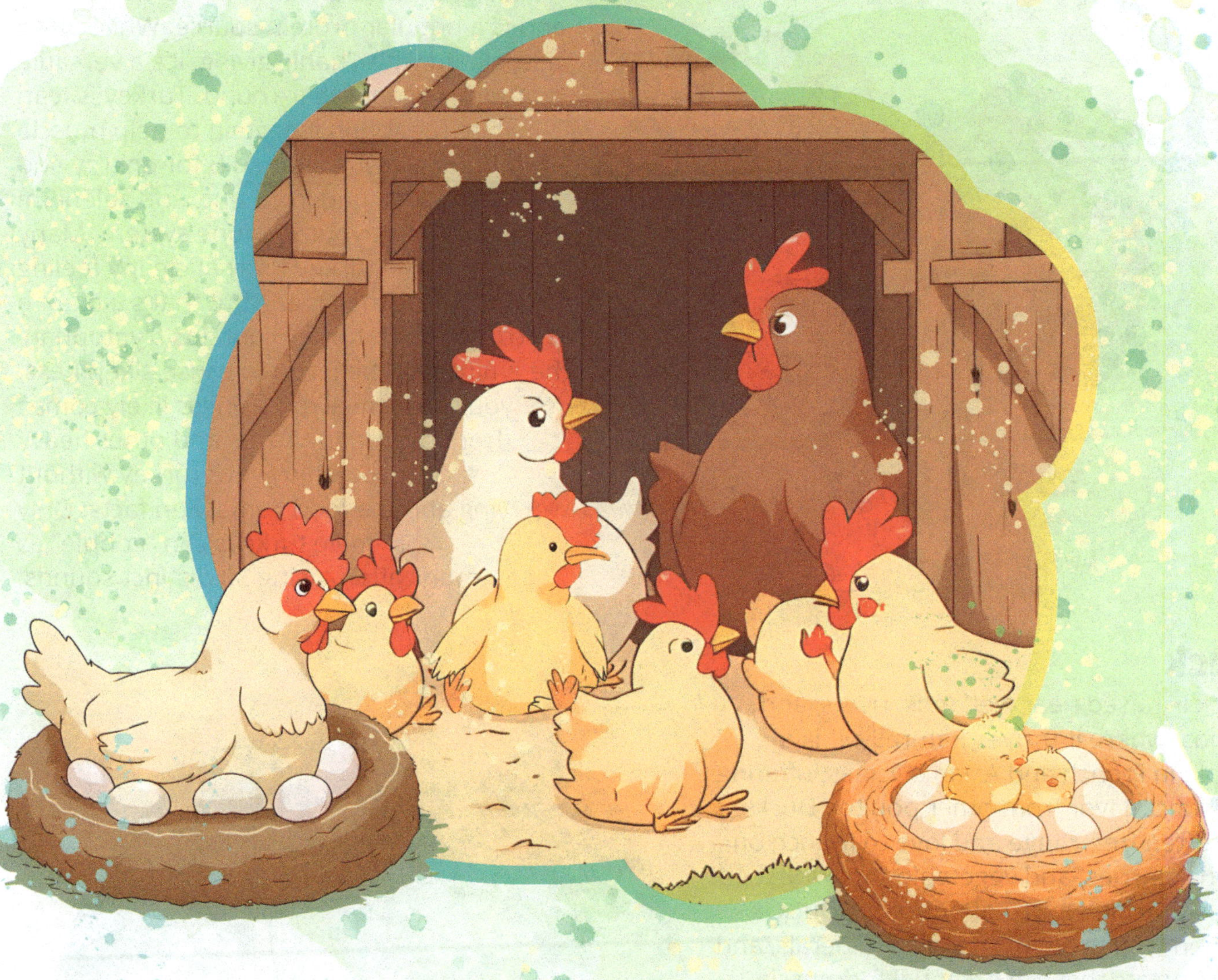

Chickens are farmed from large commercial farms to small family homesteads and have become a huge part of our food supply in a growing population and a staple in numerous cuisines. Compared to other meats, chicken offers lean protein, vitamins A and B, phosphorus, and selenium, which are important for muscle growth and recovery. Chicken also provides eggs, which are an essential food supply with high nutritional benefits. Chickens show the same Rapid Eye Movement (REM) sleep as humans, which is when dreaming happens. Ironically, the ancient Romans used chickens to predict the future. No wonder they always look sleepy, probably dreaming of the future.

Turkey

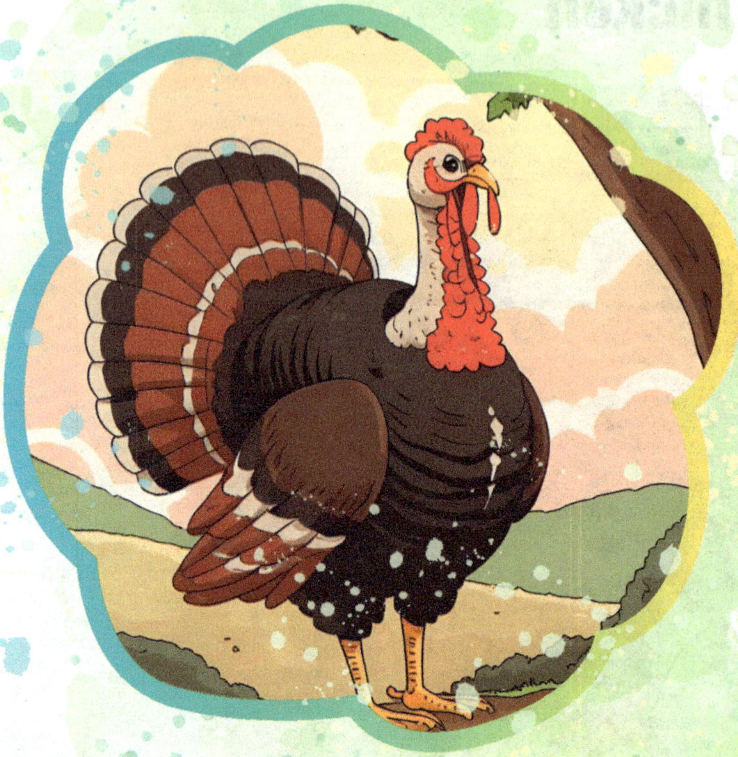

This social bird is native to North America and is a popular protein source. While often associated with Thanksgiving, it's a versatile food available year-round. Turkey is lean white meat full of protein to help muscle and brain growth, vitamin B for energy and mood boost, and iron, zinc, and selenium that support your immune system. Many people blame turkey for that sleepy feeling after a big holiday meal, but that's a bit of a myth. Although turkey contains tryptophan, the amino acid believed to cause sleepiness, your post-meal drowsiness likely comes from overeating carbs and other heavy foods. So enjoy your turkey without worrying about a food coma. Fun facts: Only male turkeys can "gobble" as communication, using 30 distinct sounds.

Duck

Duck is raised near wetlands, rivers, and ponds, where it thrives naturally. It is a staple in French and Asian cuisines, offering a distinct flavor from other poultry. Ducks are often free-range and love to munch on seeds, berries, and vegetables, making them a sustainable source of nutrients. Duck is loaded with protein, vitamins, minerals, and healthy fats that are essential for muscle building and strong bones. In fact, the darker "red meat" portion of duck contains more myoglobin, giving it a richer color and higher iron content than chicken or turkey. Duck also has a unique low-melting-point fat that can be rendered out during cooking, leaving behind a rich, bold oil great for frying and a leaner, crispy piece of meat.

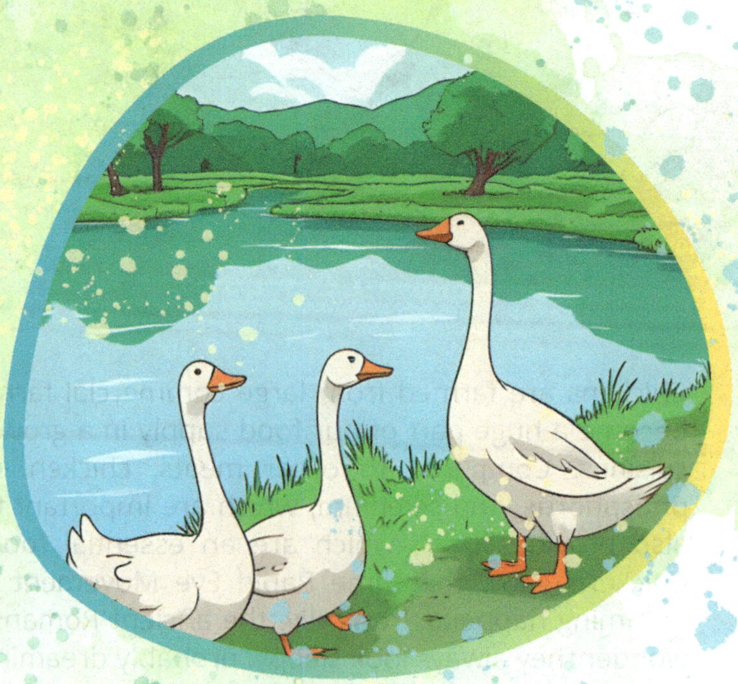

Ostrich

Ostriches, which live in the hot savannah of Africa, are primarily omnivores and can lay the world's biggest eggs. These tall birds have eyes bigger than their brain, giving them excellent vision to run faster than any other birds at speeds of up to 45 miles per hour. Despite its unpopularity as the main source of poultry, ostrich scored the highest for overall nutrient density, making it the healthiest choice of protein among other poultry that is rich in iron, vitamin B, phosphorus, and low in fat and cholesterol. These nutrients are essential for energy sources, building muscle, bones, and teeth, and a healthy nervous system. Its nutritional benefits make it a good fit for some diets and for those seeking lower-calorie and easily digestible options.

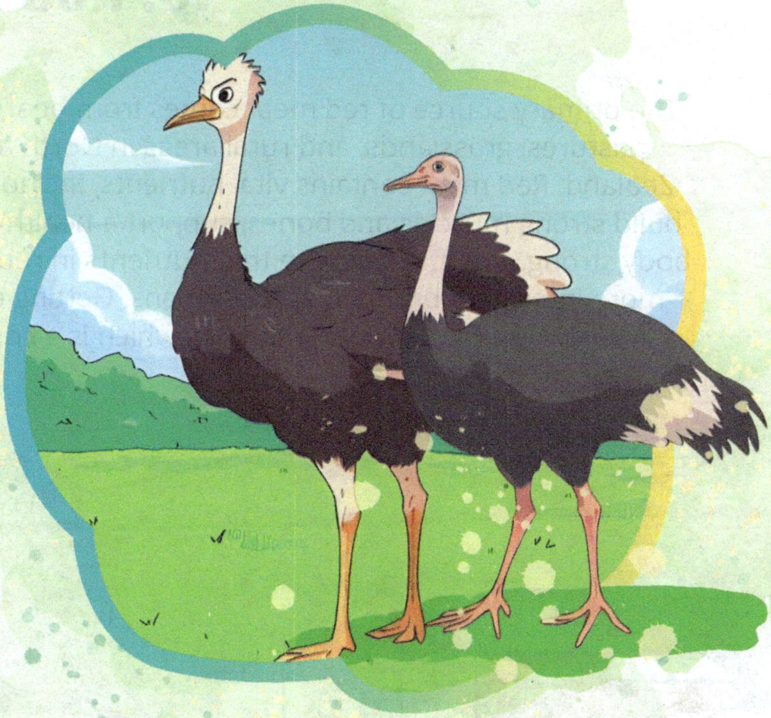

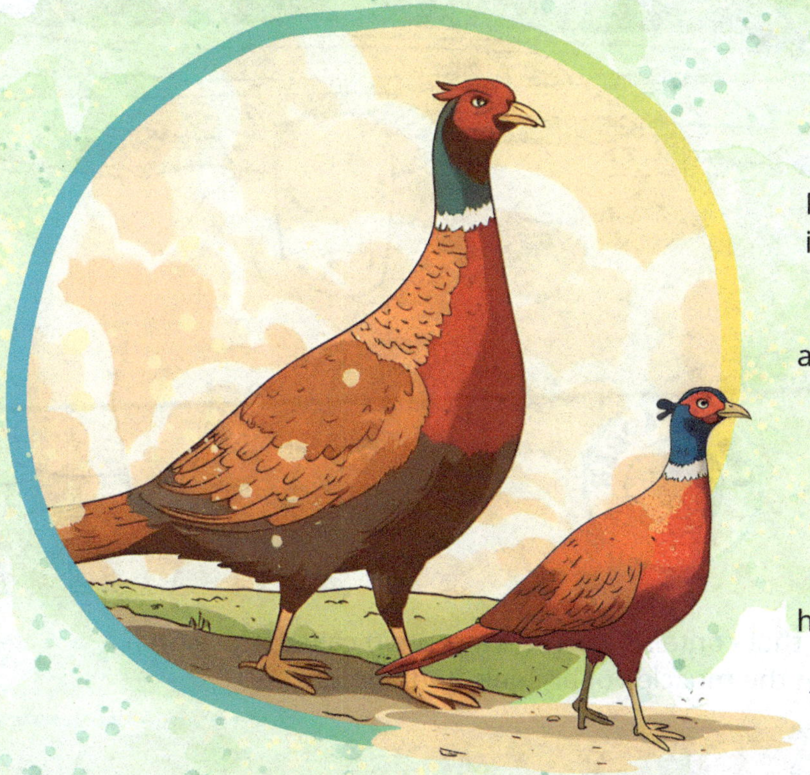

Pheasant

Pheasants are beautiful wild birds found in grasslands and farmlands across Asia, Europe, and North America. They prefer open landscapes with a blend of fields and forests that offer food and a place to live. Historically, they've been a popular game bird, but now they are raised on farms for food. Pheasant meat is rich in lean protein, vitamins B6 and B12, essential for muscle growth and recovery, support nerve function, and a healthy immune system. Pheasants are a good choice for lean protein because they have less fat than other poultry. It's a real win-win for your plate.

10. Red Meats

The primary source of red meat comes from beef, lamb, pork, and venison raised on farms, open pastures, grasslands, and rural areas in North and South America, China, Australia, and New Zealand. Red meat contains vital nutrients, including protein, iron, zinc, and vitamins, which help build strong muscles and bones, support a healthy brain as you grow, boost energy, and keep the body strong. Scientists believe that nutrients in red meat contributed to the development of larger, more intelligent brains in early humans. Getting enough red meat helps prevent and treat iron-deficiency anemia, which is a common issue for many people.

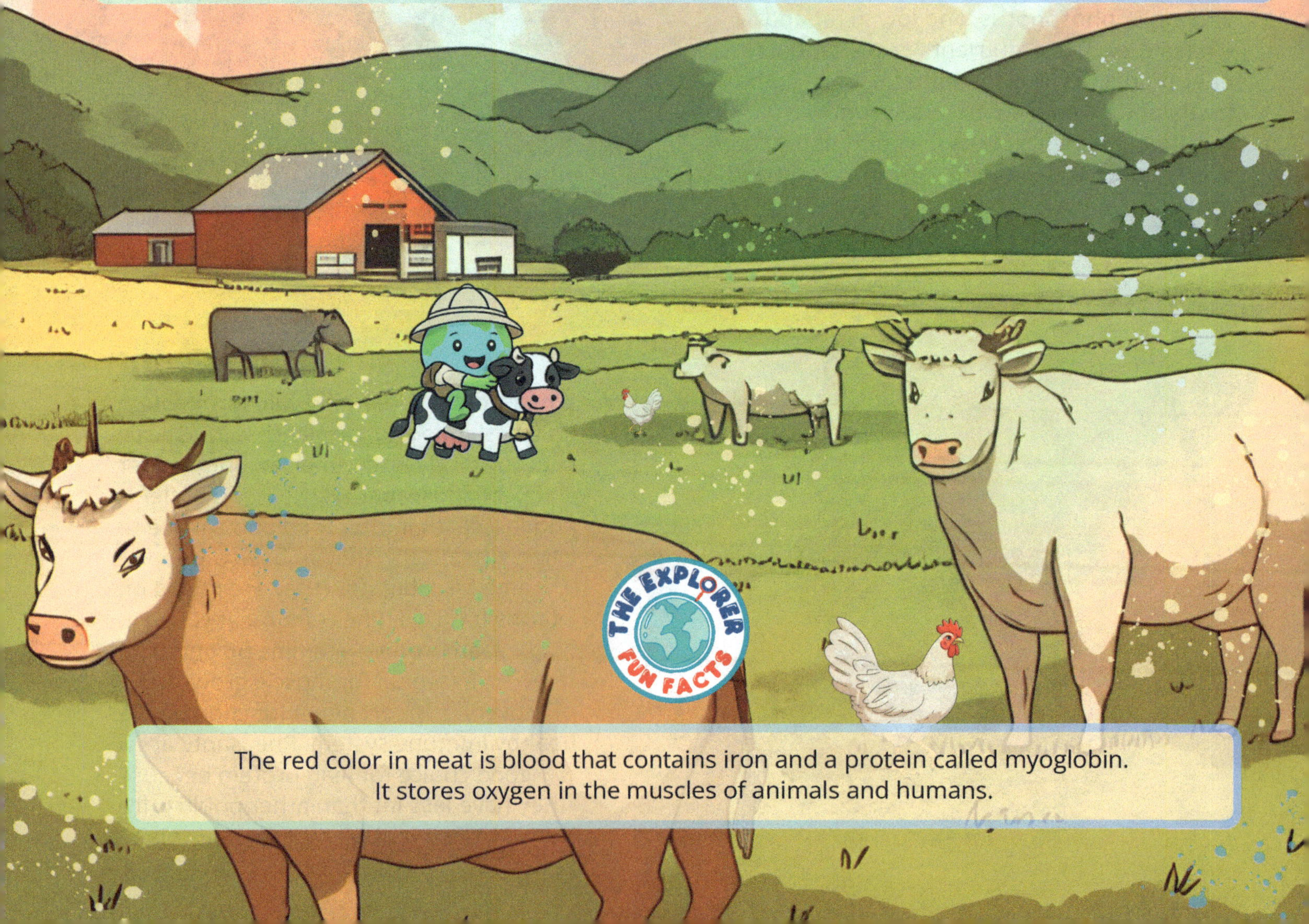

The red color in meat is blood that contains iron and a protein called myoglobin. It stores oxygen in the muscles of animals and humans.

Beef

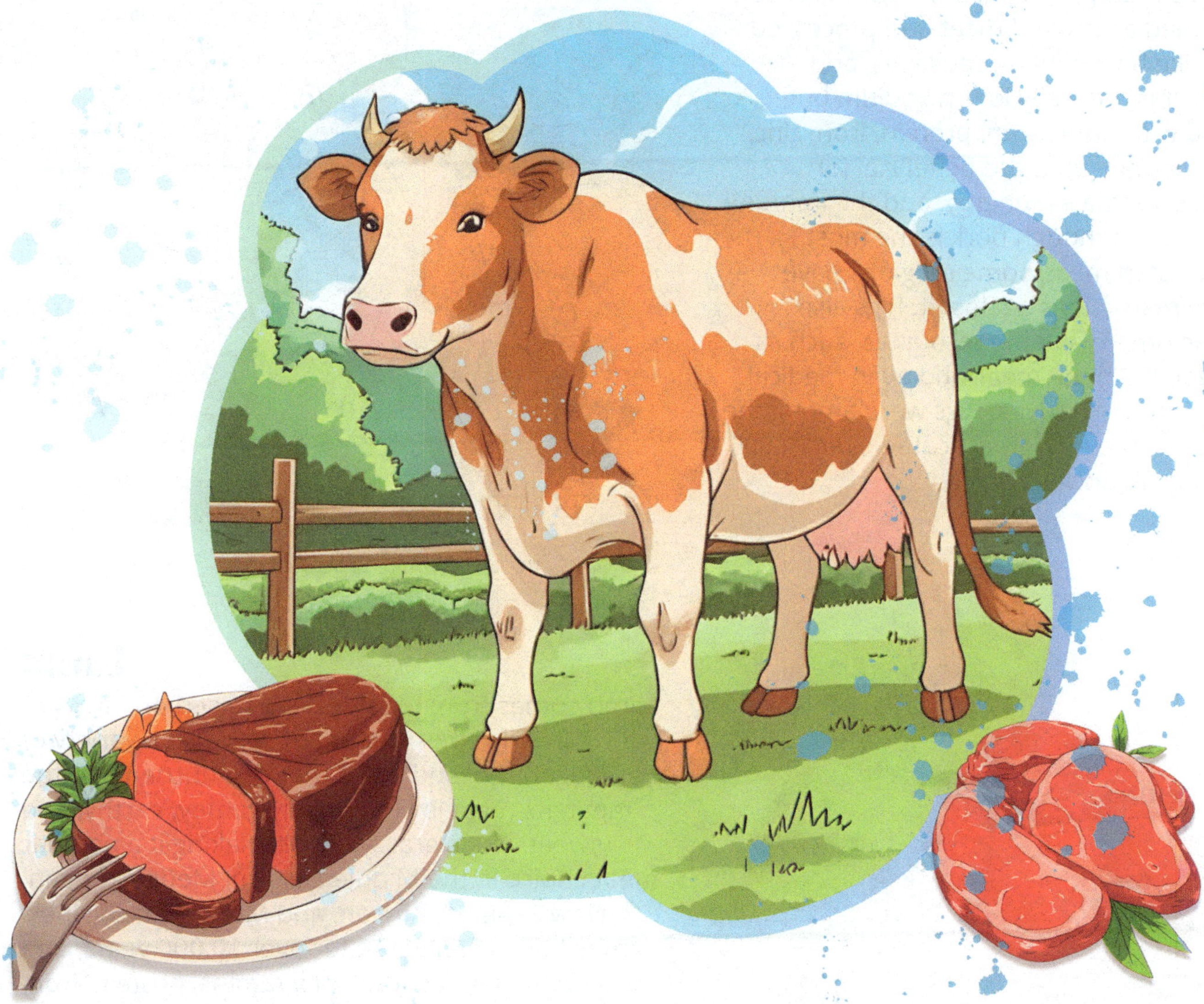

Beef comes from cattle raised in open grasslands or pastures in North and South America, Australia, and Europe. Cows have a four-compartment stomach that helps them break down tough grasses and plants that humans can't eat and convert into nutritious food for us. It contains 10 essential nutrients that support growth, brain development, energy levels, immunity, and overall body health. One serving of beef can give the body all the essential amino acids it needs. Cattle also provide several valuable by-products, including leather and medications.

Pork

Pork is a food product from pigs. It is widely consumed as cooked meat and processed foods like bacon, ham, sausages, and salami. It is naturally low in sodium but packed with potassium, protein, iron, zinc, and B vitamins that are beneficial for muscles, increased energy, and the immune system. Even though pork is the most widely eaten meat, some religions have dietary restrictions against it. Pigs also provide other valuable resources, such as lard, gelatin, bone meal, and even medical items like heart valves. Pigs were among the first animals ever domesticated over 10,000 years ago in ancient China.

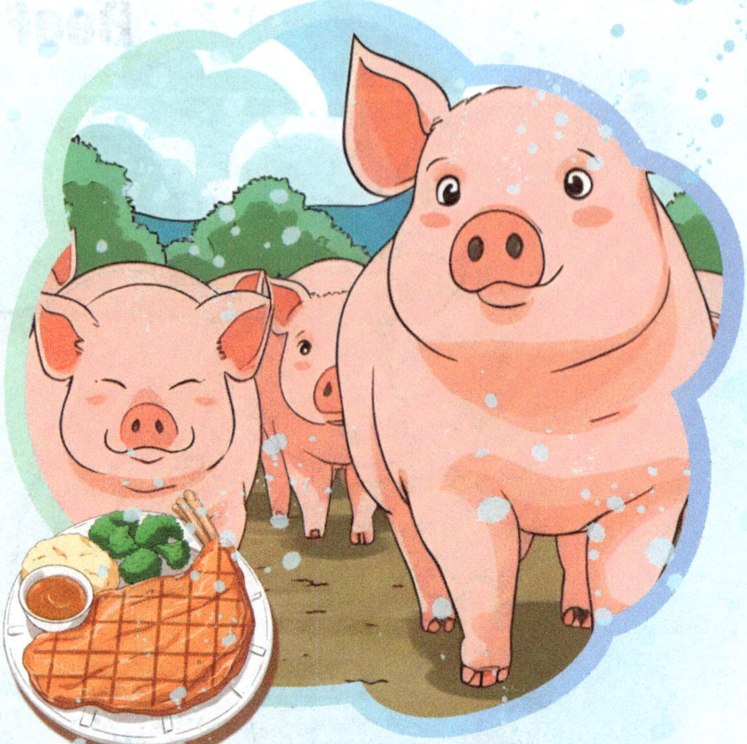

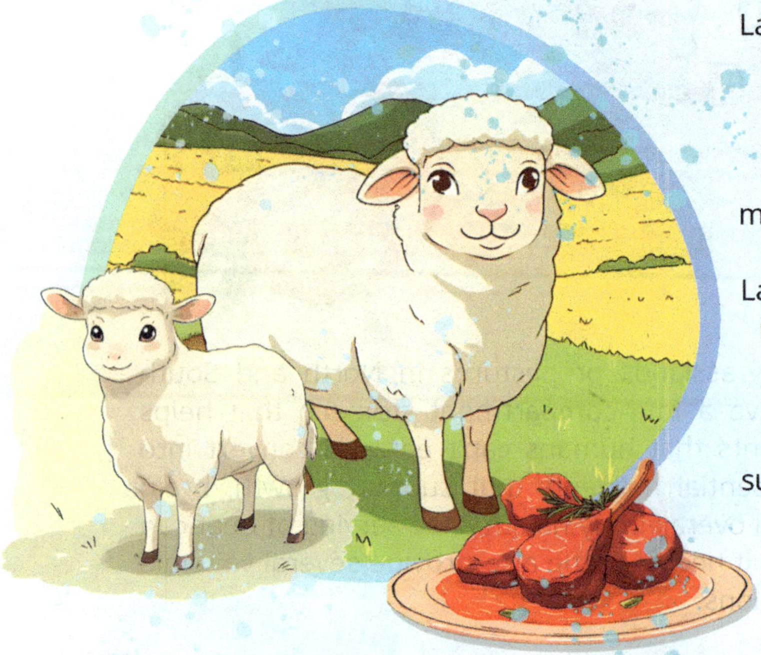

Lamb

Lamb comes from young sheep raised on farms or in hilly open pasture, grazing on a variety of vegetation and grass that add nutrients to the meat. Its meat is distinctively gamey, earthy, and sweet with a grassy flavor, making it a popular meat choice in the Middle Eastern, Mediterranean, New Zealand, African, and Mongolian cuisines. Lambs have been eaten for over 10,000 years, and it is an excellent source of vitamins, protein, iron, and zinc. These nutrients help reduce bad cholesterol in the blood, lower the risk of heart disease, increase red blood cell production, support immunity, and enhance healing functions. The unique thing about lambs is that they have rectangular pupils that give 360-degree vision to spot predators and the ability to recognize their mother’s sound as a way of communication.

Venison

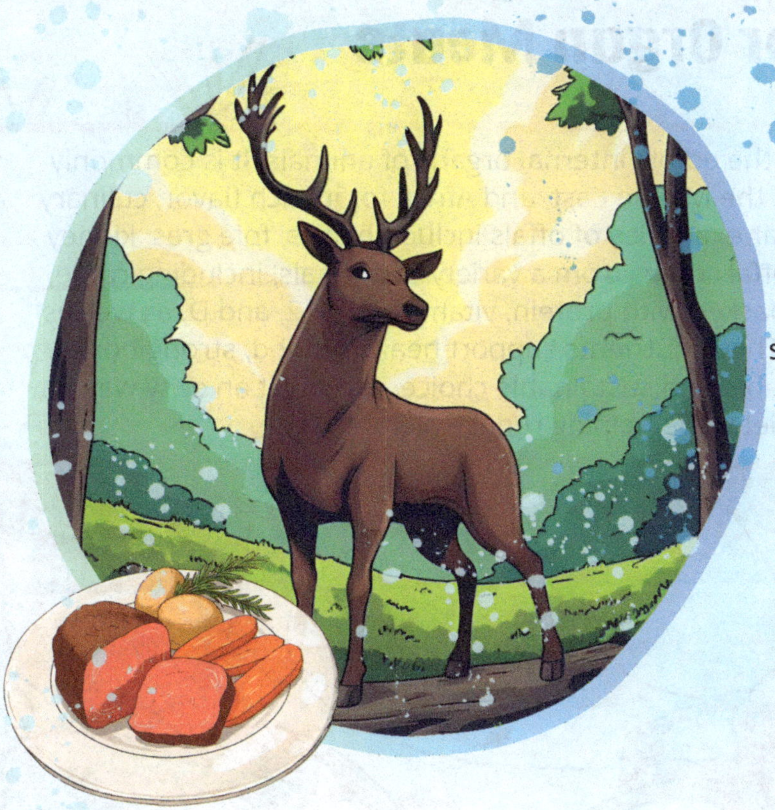

Venison is a culinary term for the meat of deer, animals known for their grace and speed. Fawns, or baby deer, are born with white spots that help them camouflage themselves in tall grass to hide from predators. Deer are herbivores that love to eat plants, grass, leaves, and flowers in the summer, and bark and branches in the winter. This natural diet adds essential nutrients to their meat, making it naturally low in fat, calories, and cholesterol. Venison is typically sourced from free-range and grass-fed farms in New Zealand. It is a high-protein meat rich in iron, vitamin B, zinc, and omega-3 fatty acids. Adding venison to your diet provides energy, supports muscle health, and helps balance your overall nutrition. In Latin, venison means "to hunt" and was considered a royal delicacy in medieval times.

Bison

Bison are fast, mighty, and the largest land mammals in North America, with males weighing up to 2,000 pounds and standing 6 feet tall. Bison are herbivores that enjoy grasses, weeds, and leafy plants, and can be found roaming the Great Plains and iconic landscapes like Yellowstone National Park. Their meat is lean and savory, with fewer calories, less fat, and rich in protein, iron, zinc, and vitamin B12 compared to beef. Bison are often raised in open, natural environments, grazing on grass and growing without added hormones. Once nearly driven to extinction, bison have made a remarkable comeback thanks to conservation efforts. Choosing bison supports sustainable farming practices and helps protect the native habitats these animals call home.

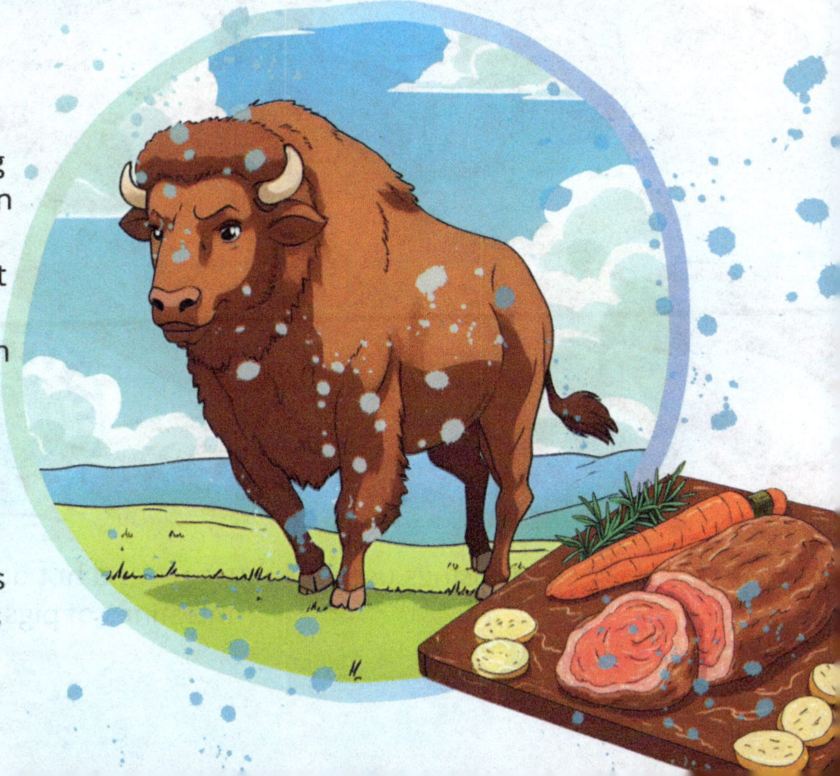

11. Offals or Organ Meats

Offal, also known as organ meats, refers to the edible internal organs of animals. It is commonly enjoyed across Europe, South America, Asia, the Middle East, and Africa for its rich flavor, culinary versatility, and high nutritional value. Popular examples of offals include haggis, foie gras, kidney pie, chicken feet, pâté, and bone marrow. Offal comes from a variety of animals, including cattle, pork, lamb, goat, chicken, and duck, and is packed with protein, vitamins A, B12, and D, as well as zinc, copper, selenium, folate, and choline. These nutrients support healthy blood, strong bones, and brain function. Offal is also an affordable and sustainable choice, making it an easy way to add variety to your daily diet while helping reduce animal waste.

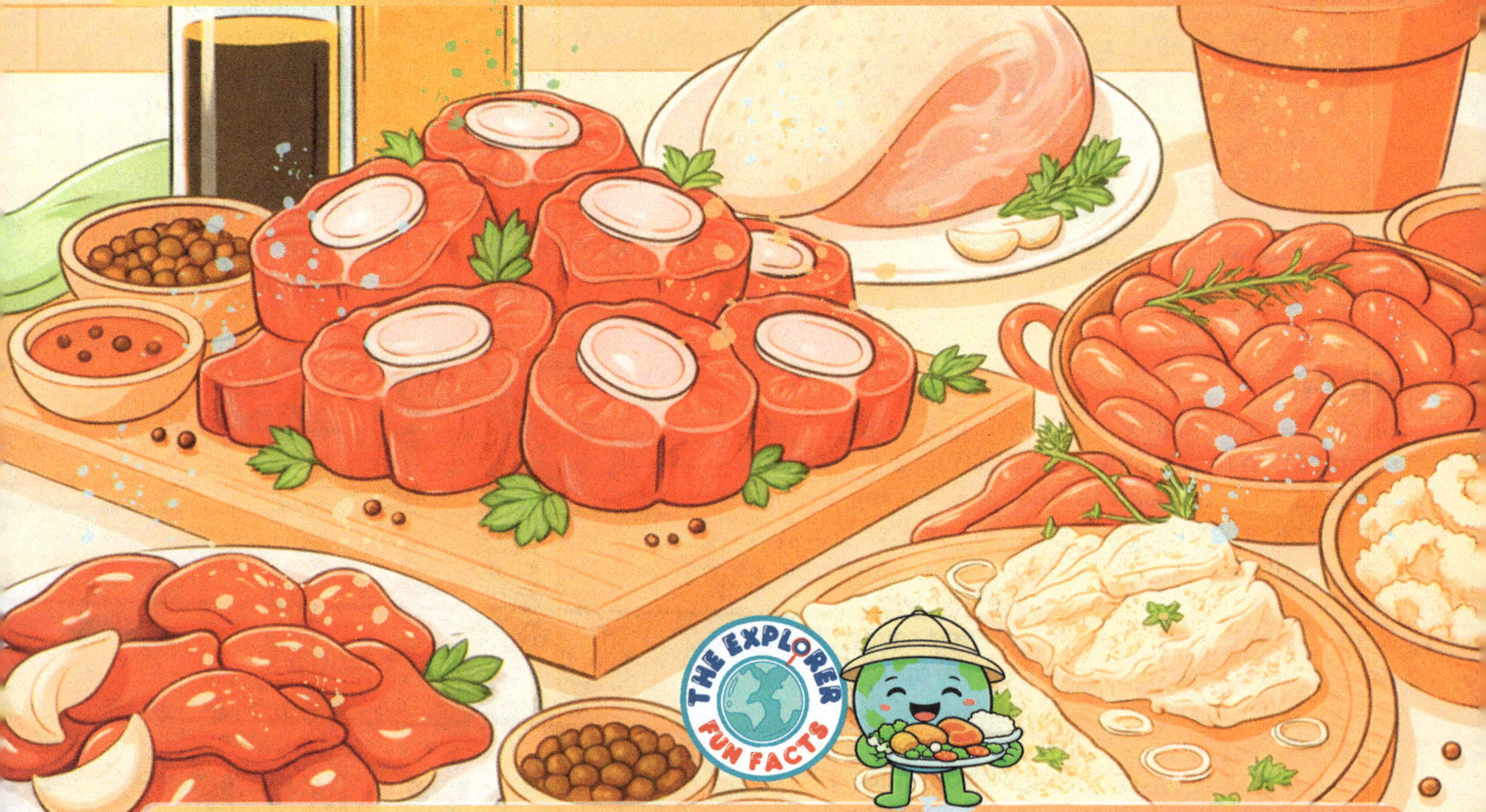

Food casings used for sausages and hot dogs are mostly made from cleaned animal intestines of pigs, sheep, or cows

Liver

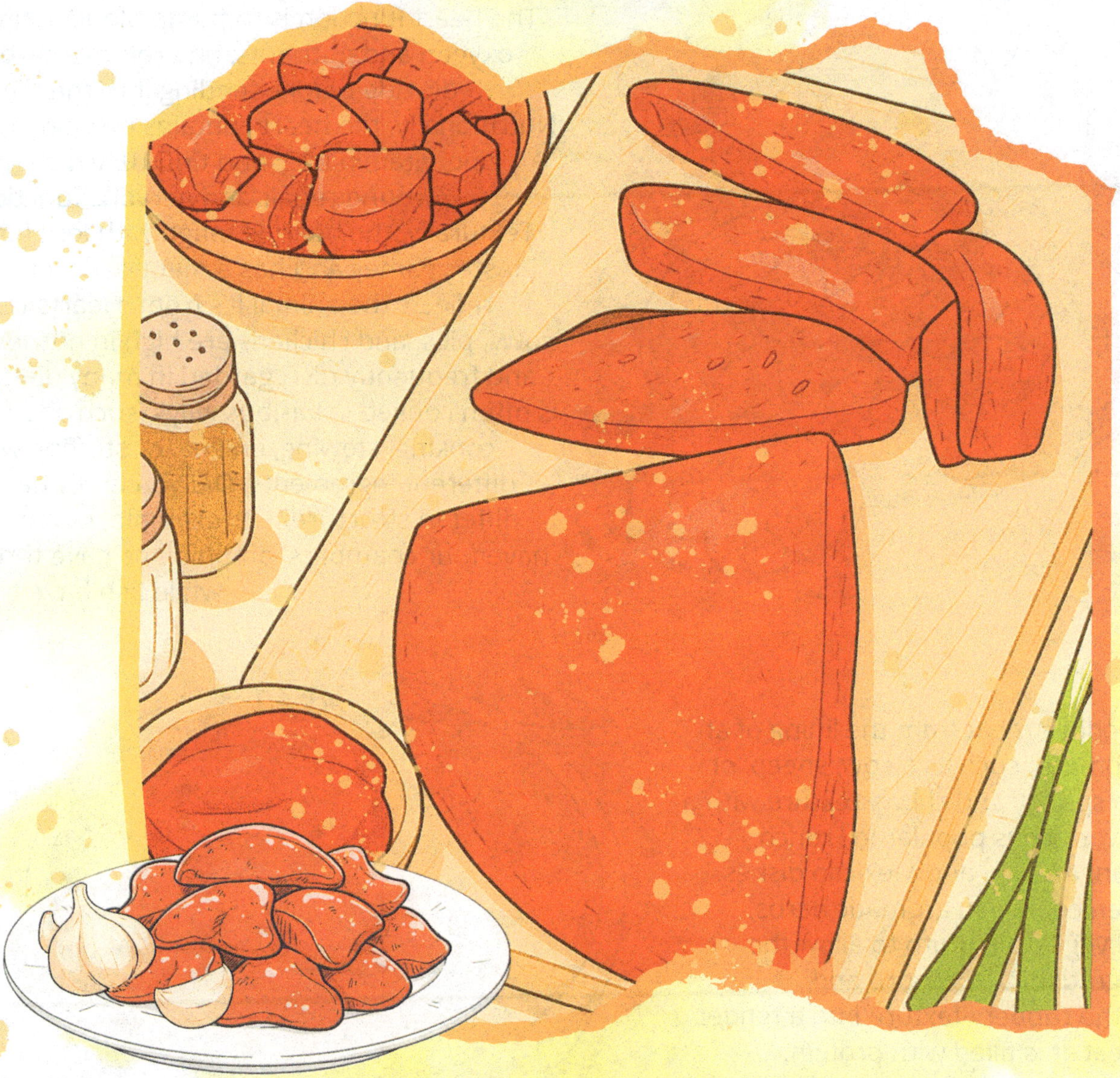

The liver cleanses the blood of toxins, breaks down food for digestion, and stores essential nutrients, vitamins, and minerals for the body's use when needed. No wonder it is a superfood in many cuisines, serving as a vital source of vitamins A, D, E, K, and B to protect against diseases. The iron, copper, and zinc content help to build muscle, enhance vision, improve brain function, and provide an energy supercharge. The liver has a special ability to regrow itself, making it a superfood rich in vitamins and minerals compared to many other food choices.

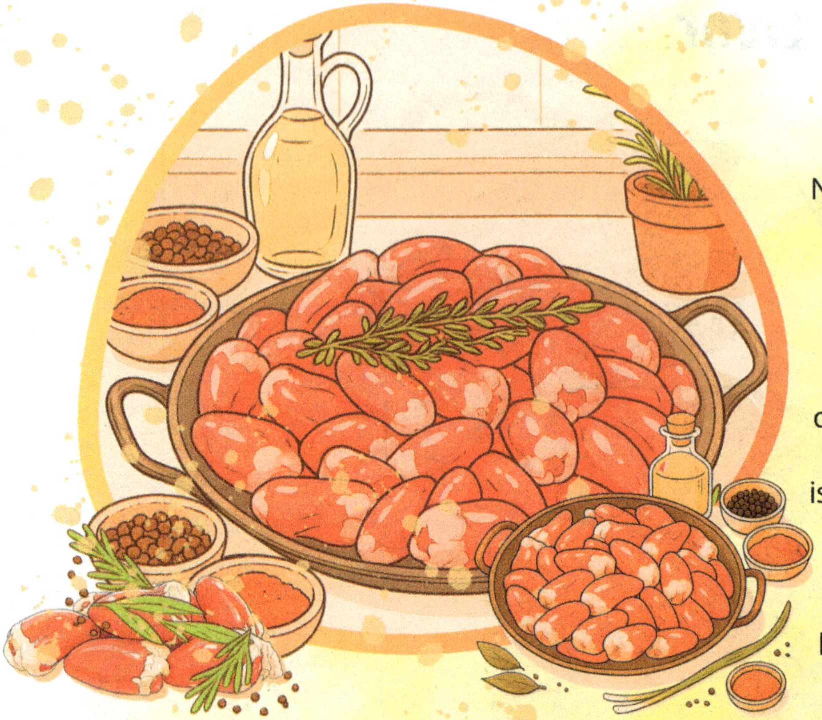

Heart

The heart function is to pump blood, deliver oxygen and nutrients, and remove carbon dioxide before sending it to the lungs. Nutritionally, the heart contains protein, iron, zinc, vitamin B12, and CoQ10, which help wound repair and nervous function. Texturally, the heart is tough with less fat. It tastes gamey and has a metallic flavor that reflects the animal it's from. Hearts from cows, pigs, and chickens are high in nutrients and frequently disregarded in many diets. It is often cooked in various ways, such as slow-cooking, stewing, grilling, or stuffing with different ingredients. Did you know hearts differ in structure? For example, mammals have four chambers, amphibians have three, while fish have two.

Tripe

Tripe is an edible meat from the lining of an animal's stomach, such as a cow, sheep, or pig. It has a spongy and chewy texture with a delicate flavor and is popular in French, Italian, Asian, African, and Mexican dishes. Tripe is often cooked in aromatic herbs, spices, and vegetable broth to allow the flavorful ingredients to absorb and transform the rubbery texture into a tender delicacy meat. It is filled with protein, vitamins, zinc, and iron, which are key for sustaining energy levels and fortifying the immune system. Tripe contains beneficial bacteria that promote a healthy gut microbiome and digestive health. Some cultures believe tripe soup is a remedy for colds and sickness.

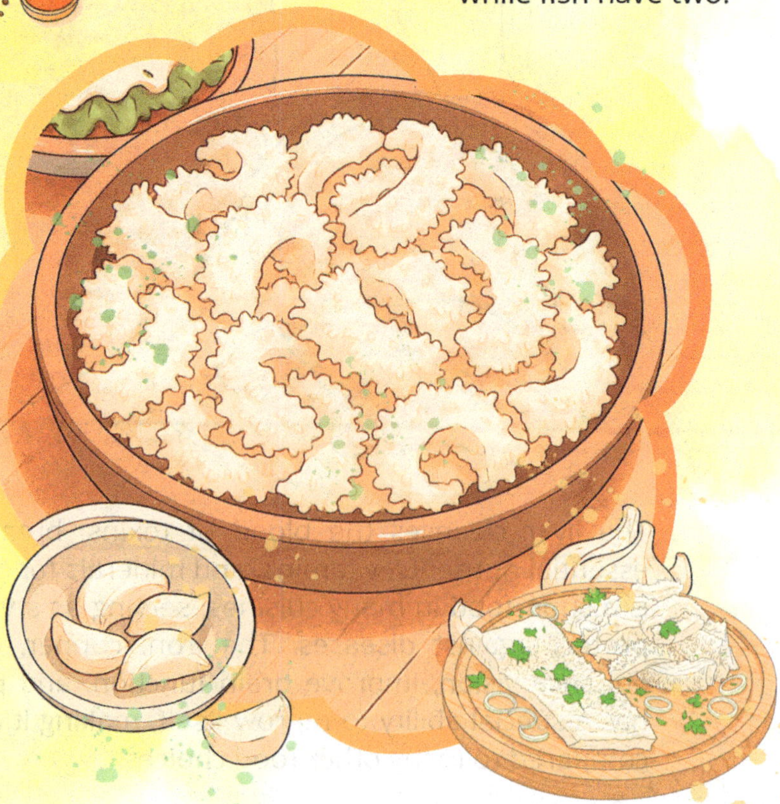

Tongue

The tongue is unique, just like a fingerprint, with different shapes, sizes, and numbers of taste buds that are unique to each person. A tongue is actually a muscle that is tender and flavorful due to its fat content, making it a delicacy in culinary because of its nutritional benefits. Beef tongue is a favorite for its high-quality protein content, fat, iron, zinc, vitamin B, and amino acids, which support muscle growth, tissue strength, hormone balance, and immune function. Cow, pig, and deer tongues are also widely served in various dishes, mostly popular in Mexican tacos and sandwiches in Eastern Europe. Similar to tripe, it requires slow cooking to tenderize the chewy muscle before the outer skin is removed before serving.

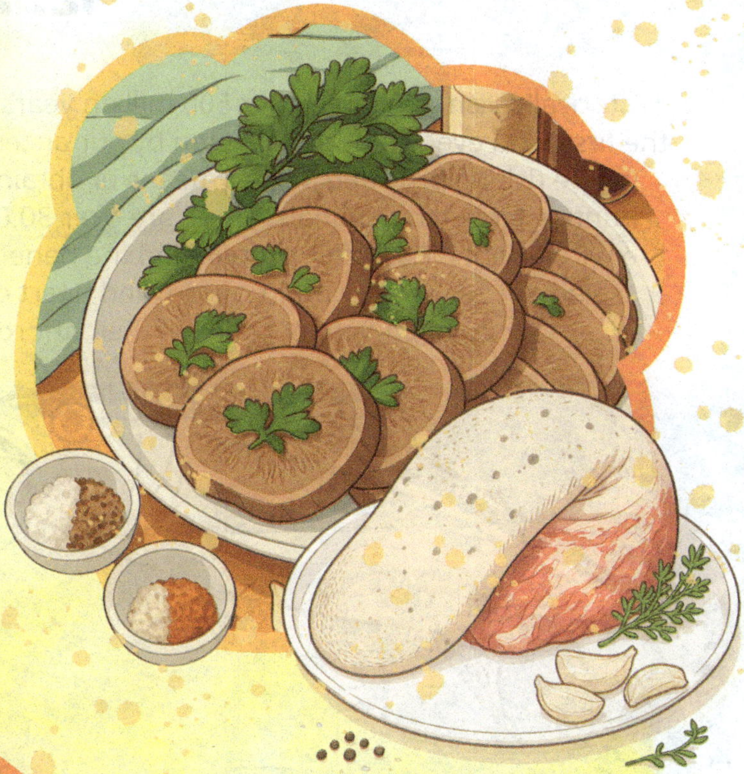

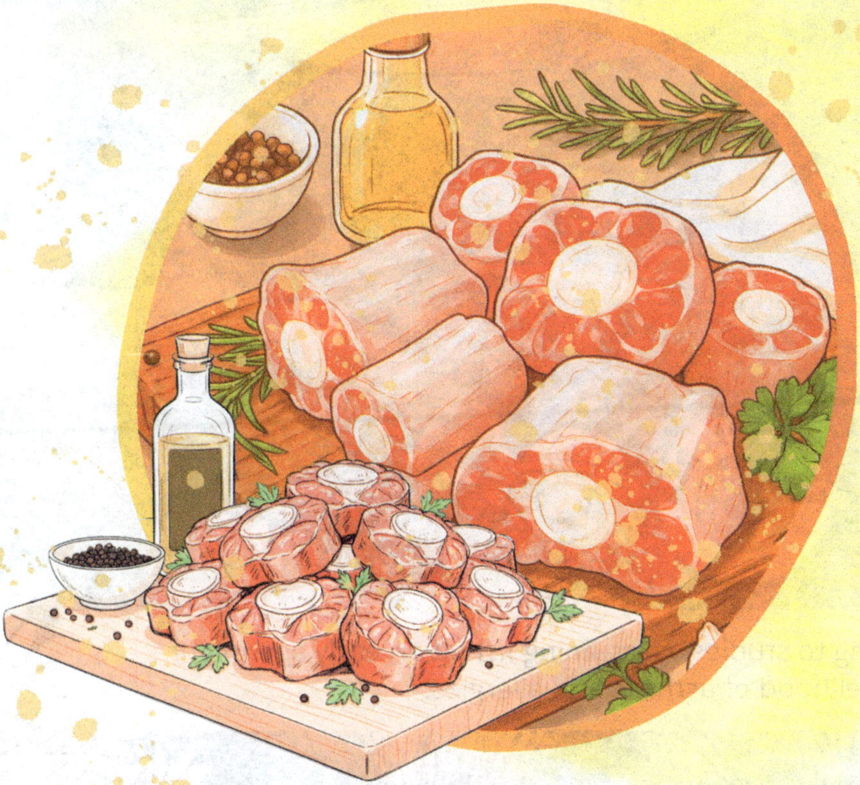

Oxtail

Oxtail comes from the tail of cattle, consumed for its beefy flavor and tender gelatinous texture. It is an affordable cut of meat rich in iron, collagen, zinc, and phosphorus, which support muscle, joint, and skin health, as well as energy production. Oxtail is traditionally a tough cut that becomes succulent and flavorful after slow cooking and is an excellent base for stews, soups, and braises. Oxtail is a popular dish in Caribbean, European, and East Asian cuisines. The long cooking process breaks down the collagen in the oxtail, which makes the gravy thick and sticky.

12. Fish

Historically, fish appeared over 500 million years ago, long before dinosaurs existed. Fish became the first food ever hunted and eaten by our ancestors. Ancient civilizations developed along rivers, where fishing provided a safer means of obtaining food compared to the risks associated with hunting large land animals. There are over 30,000 fish species, and they live in various aquatic environments. Fish offer protein and the beneficial omega-3 fatty acids, vitamin D, iodine, and selenium needed for brain, vision, and heart development. Nowadays, salmon and tuna are popular choices because of their affordability and versatility in many cuisines.

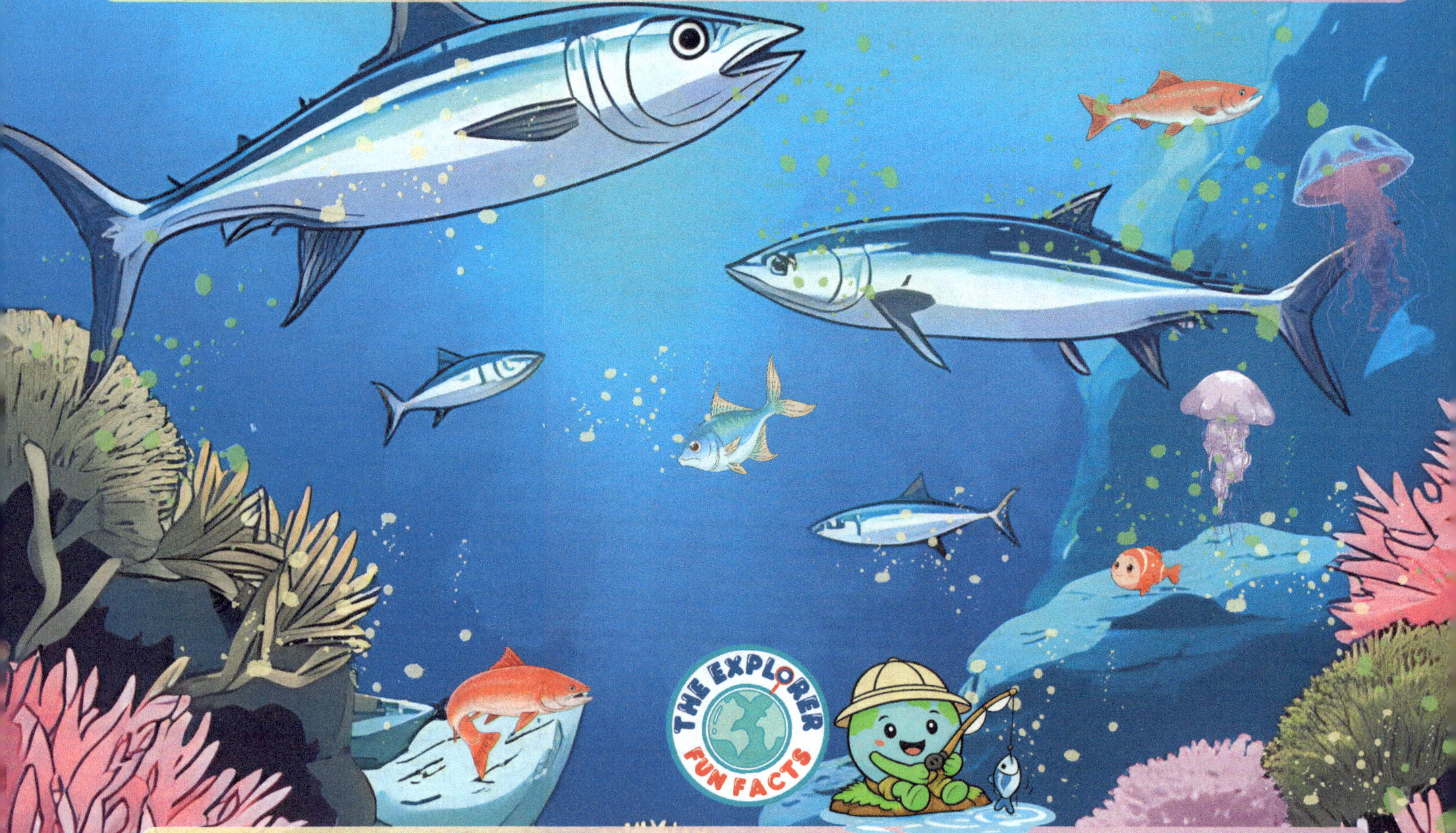

Fish is an allergy fighter. According to studies, consuming fish at an early age might reduce the likelihood of asthma and allergies.

Salmon

According to historical evidence, salmon was part of the Neanderthals' diet dating back over 200,000 years ago. It was also a sacred food and staple in many Indigenous cultures. In the wild, salmon use magnetic fields and smell to navigate back to the exact river where they were born to lay eggs. Salmon can leap over 6 feet, travel miles through the ocean, and swim upstream. They change colors from silver to vibrant red, green, or brown as they move between saltwater and freshwater. It's not surprising they are a great source of protein, omega-3s, like DHA, and vitamin D. These nutrients are super important for brain and eye development, helping kids grow strong and healthy. Salmon has a mild, delicious taste that is great served grilled, fried into nuggets, or mixed in pasta.

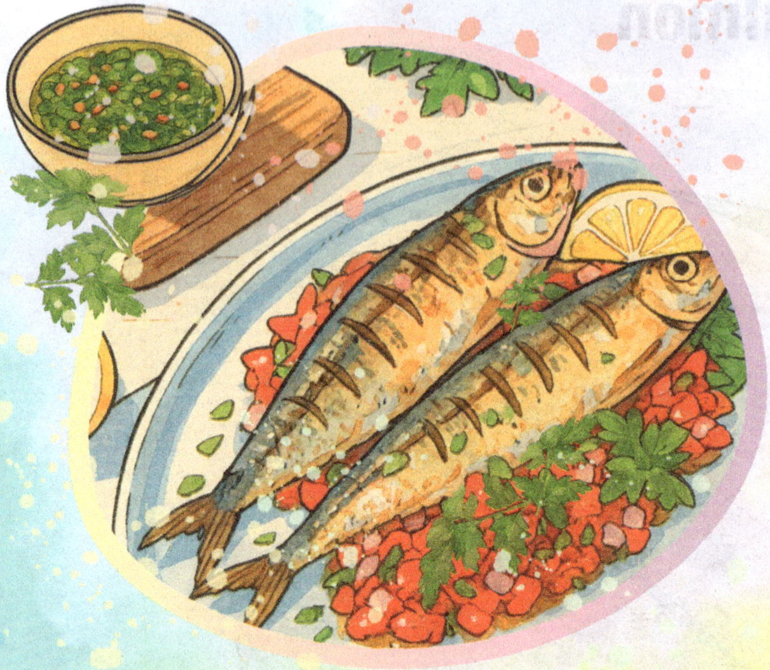

Sardine

Sardines are tiny oily fish thriving in clean coastal waters around Europe, North Africa, and the Pacific Ocean. Named after the Sardinian island, where it was once abundant, it is actually a member of the herring family. Sardines can be enjoyed fresh or grilled, rich in omega-3 fatty acids, protein, calcium, vitamin D, and B12, which are great for heart, brain, and bone health. It's commonly preserved in cans and is easy to enjoy all year round. Canned sardines, which come with soft edible bones, are an excellent source of calcium, supporting strong bones and teeth. Sardines have earned the nickname "superfish" are a sustainable seafood because of their plankton diet and low mercury content.

Tuna

Tuna are fast swimmers, capable of reaching speeds faster than most cars, at 40 miles per hour. They live in the warm Pacific and Atlantic oceans. Bluefin species can grow very large, weighing up to 2,000 pounds, and can raise their body temperature to swim long distances in a wide range of temperatures and speeds. No wonder it is a powerful source of protein, healthy fats, vitamin D, iron, and selenium that help build muscles and keep us feeling full and strong. Tuna tastes differently depending on the species, from the light albacore's creamy and buttery flavor to the more intense flavor of the yellowfin species. The classic way of enjoying tuna is in a tuna sandwich, grilled, or in sushi.

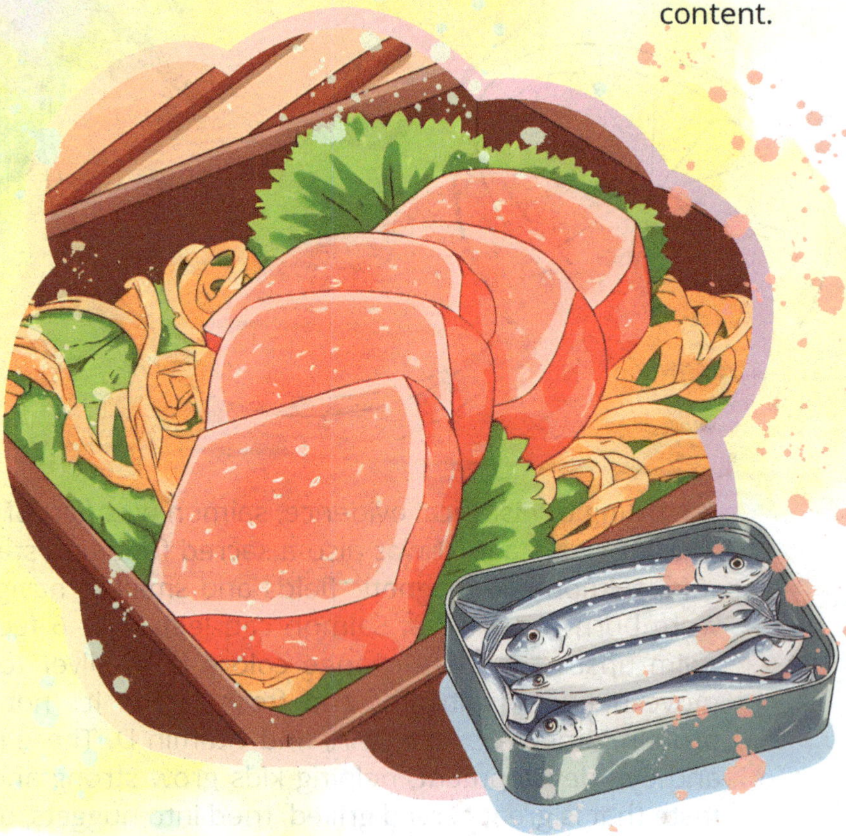

Herring

Herring are small with silvery scales, often growing to about 10 to 12 inches long. They are a huge part of the marine food found in temperate waters in the North Atlantic and Pacific Ocean. A female herring can lay 200,000 eggs, making them a key food source for bigger fish, seabirds, and marine mammals, but also a nutritional powerhouse for us. They are part of Northern Europe and Scandinavia's favorite cuisine, typically salted, smoked, or pickled in brines, served at the New Year for good luck. Herring are so oily that they were once used to fuel lamps. Now they fuel healthy diets that are rich in protein, omega-3 fatty acids, vitamin D, and B12, essential for heart, brain, and bone health.

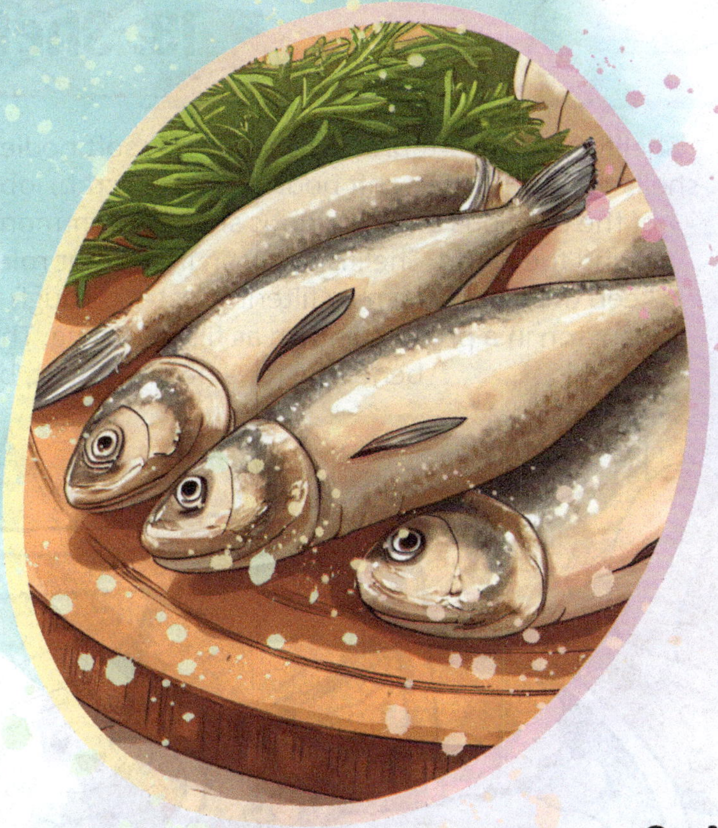

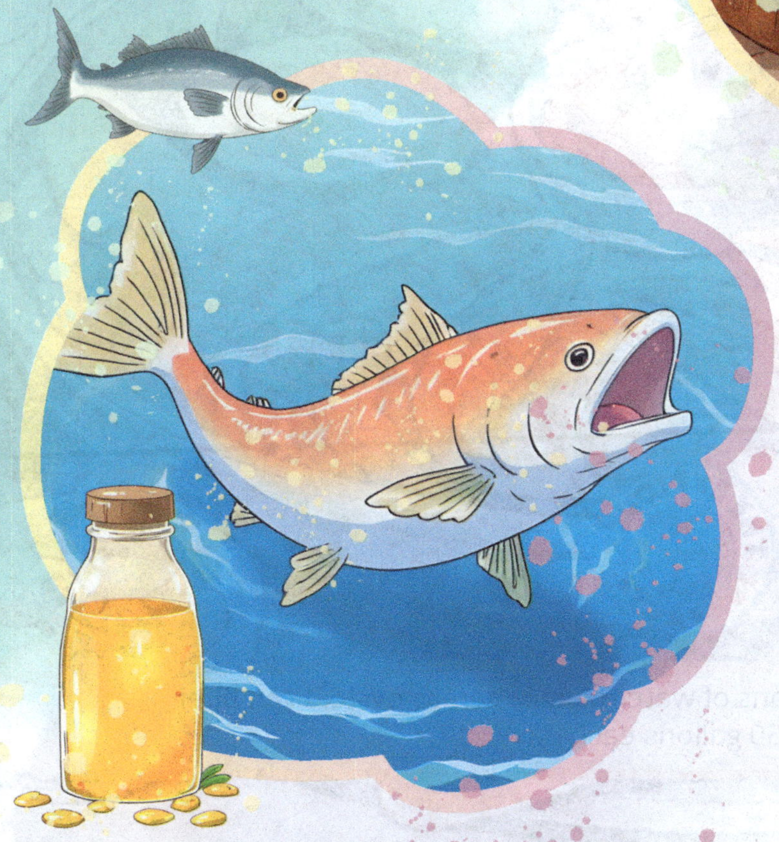

Cod

Cod thrive in the cold and deep sea waters of the Arctic and the North Atlantic Oceans. For centuries, it has been an important food, fueling the Vikings and the explorers at sea. Cod was dried and salted, making it last a long time on long sea voyages. This white fish has lean and a mild flavor loaded with omega-3, vitamin B12, and iodine, which are vital for the brain's growth, a healthy immune system, and the development of strong bones. Cod is a low-mercury fish, making it safe to eat. For centuries, cod liver oil has been a popular remedy and a source of vitamins A and D to promote immune system health and prevent serious bone diseases.

13. Shellfish

Shellfish are invertebrates that possess soft bodies and lack of bones. Many shellfish grow hard shells to protect their soft bodies. Shrimp, crab, lobster, clams, mussels, and oysters are examples of the delicious and nutritious shellfish commonly found in oceans, bays, and coastal waters around the world. Shellfish play an important role in marine food chains and ecosystems. They keep the ocean clean by filtering water through their gills to catch food, particles, algae, and plankton in a process known as filter feeding. They are rich in minerals and fat, making them beneficial for a healthy heart, brain, and immune system.

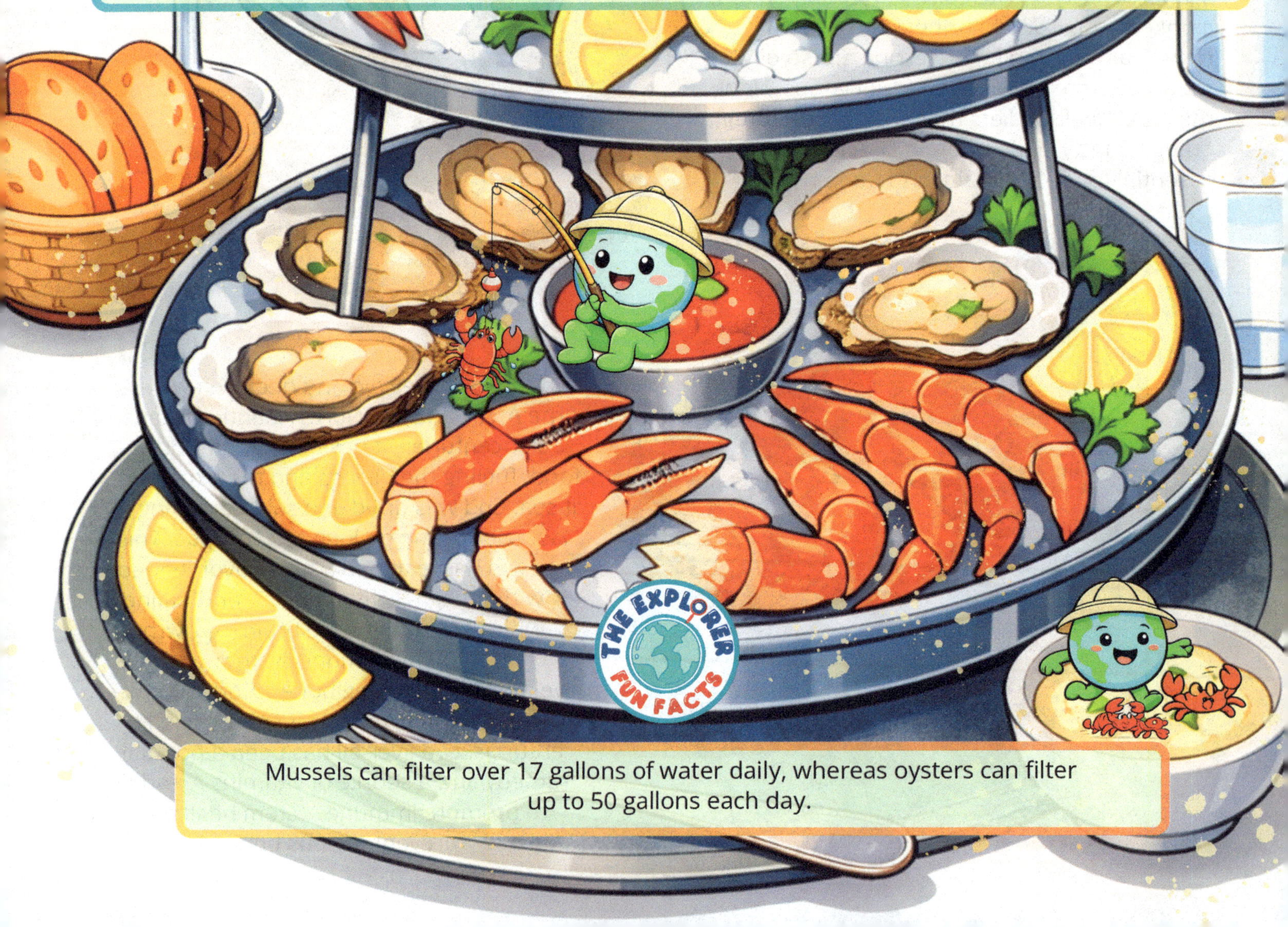

Mussels can filter over 17 gallons of water daily, whereas oysters can filter up to 50 gallons each day.

Oyster

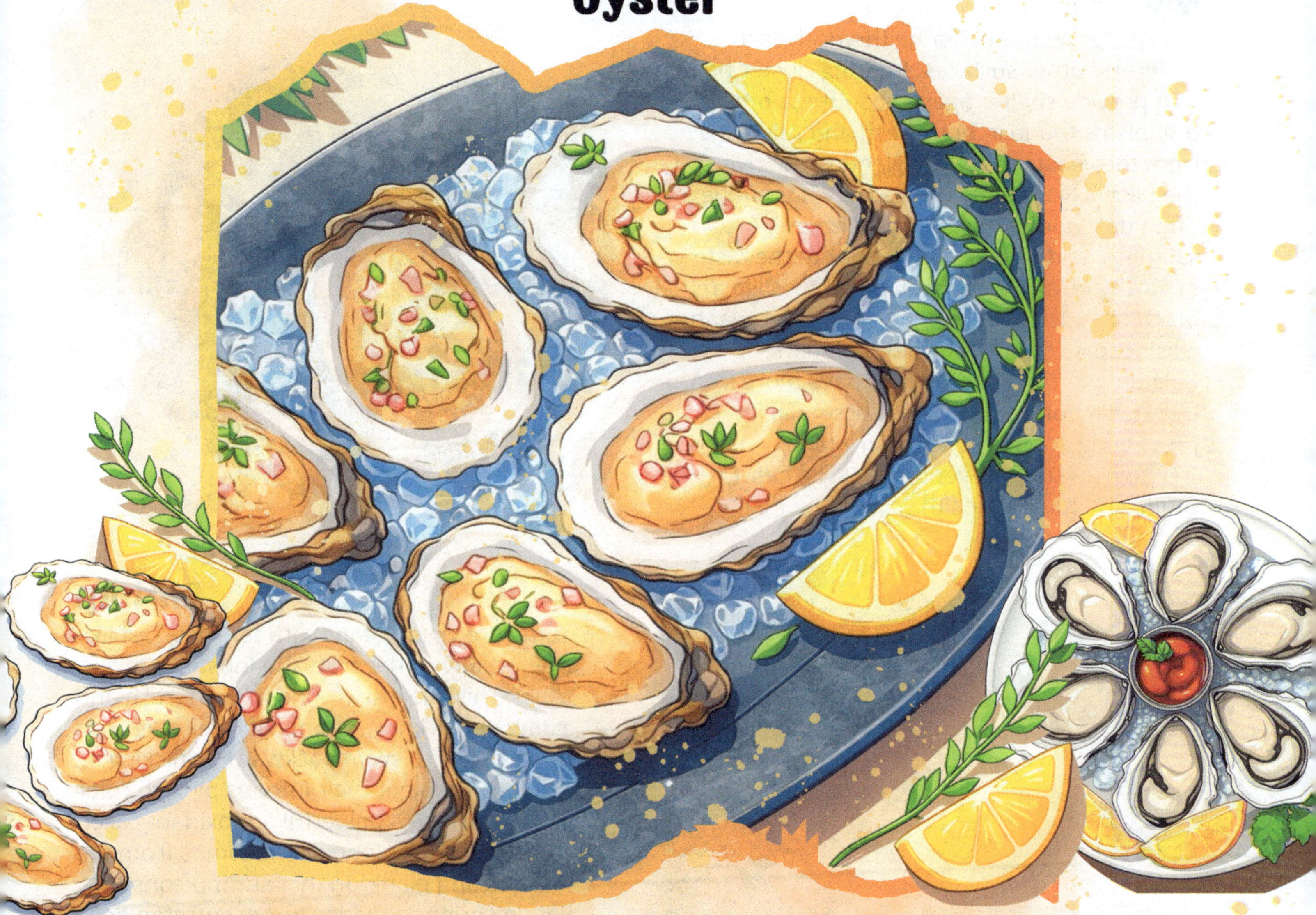

This unique filter feeder shellfish can actually change its gender back and forth from female to male to help with reproduction and population growth. Most oysters are born as males and transform into females in their first year. Changes in reef conditions, food supplies, water temperature, and the chemistry of its environment can trigger the gender changes. Regardless of its gender, both male and female oysters can produce pearls. This unique shellfish accumulates high zinc content to support its own immunity, which means consuming oysters helps us build a strong immune system and enhances our sense of taste and smell. These delicacies are low in calorie content but high in protein and vitamin B12, which is beneficial to our healthy brain, bones, and energy.

Mussel

Mussels grow by anchoring themselves to rocks and other surfaces, forming cluster beds that provide shelter against countless other organisms found in both fresh and salt water from the coasts of New England to the rivers of the Pacific Northwest. Mussel flavor is subtle, often described as a mix of sweetness, saltiness, and tenderness, similar to the taste of earthy mushrooms, and it cooks well in a broth or sauce. They are popular in European cuisine, particularly in Spain, Denmark, Belgium, and France. Mussels have more iron than a fillet of steak, which is essential for preventing anemia. It is rich in vitamins A and B12 to help support your eyes, skin, heart, brain, and muscle health.

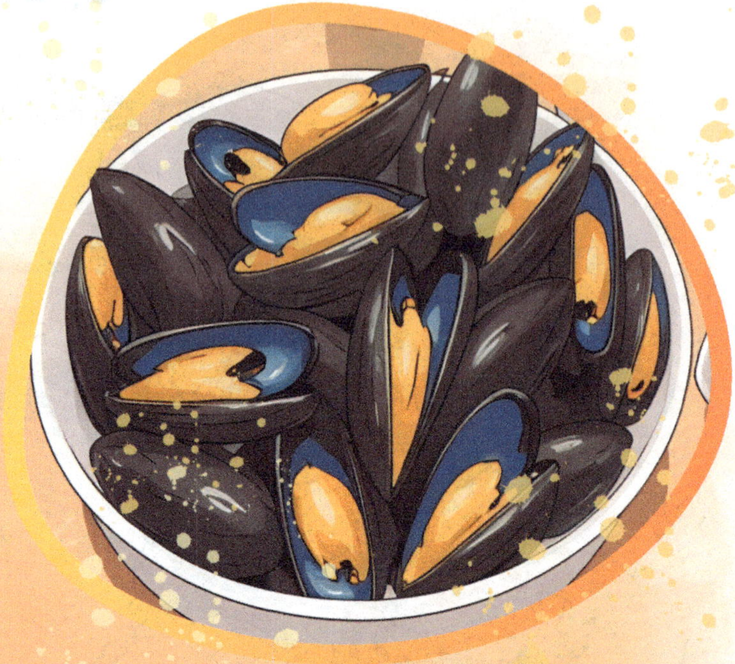

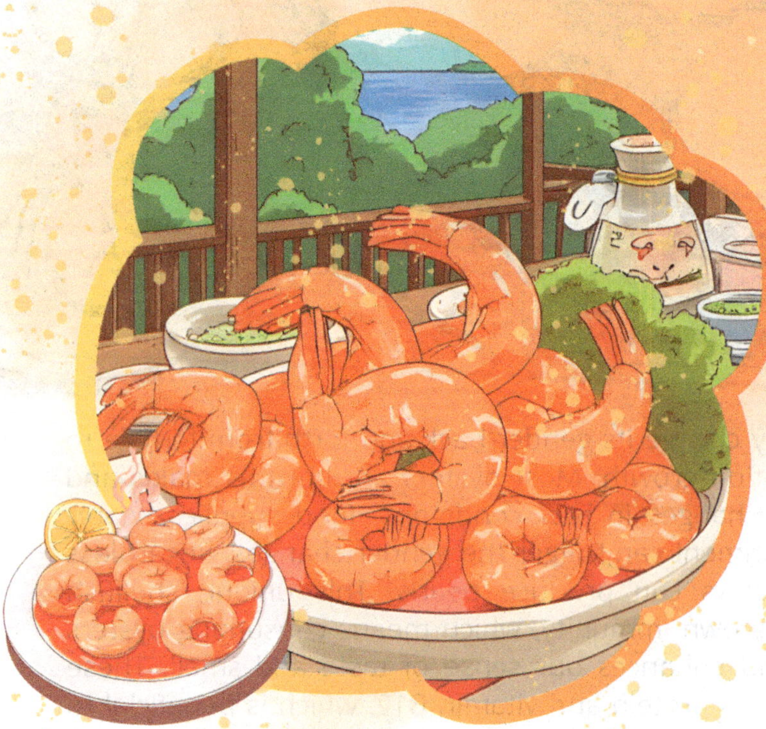

Shrimp

Shrimp are crustaceans with ten legs, just like their relatives, the crab and lobster families. This shellfish, found in both fresh and saltwater, is known for its hard exoskeleton and its ability to swim backward by flicking its tail. Shrimp get their famous pinkish color from a powerful antioxidant called astaxanthin. This antioxidant comes from the algae and plankton that shrimp consume. Eating shrimp provides a concentrated dose of that same beneficial compound. Shrimp is a delicacy that has been a staple since ancient Roman and Greek times. It can be cooked in various ways, such as being dried, fermented, or salted. Shrimp is small, low in fat and calories, but mighty in nutrients, helping with energy, immunity, and nerve function.

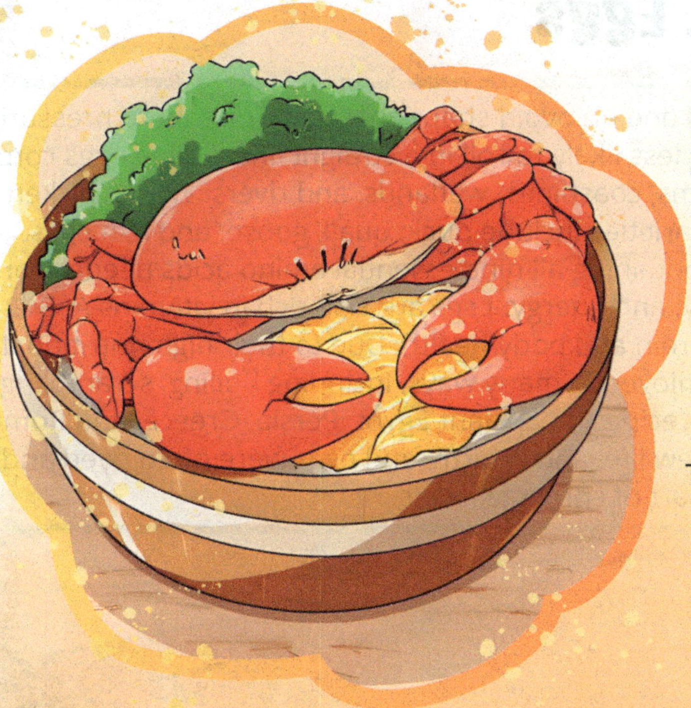

Crab

Archaeological evidence suggests that crabs were part of the Neanderthal diet over 90,000 years ago. It later became a food source for the Greeks, Romans, Chinese, Japanese, and Native Americans in the coastal regions where they were easily found. Crab is typically roasted and boiled for its savory taste, a combination of sweet and salty notes reminiscent of the sea, and features a firm yet soft texture. Crabs are omnivores, feeding on algae, small fish, other crustaceans, and decaying plants or animals. This diet provides crab meat that is packed with iron, omega-3, and vitamin B1, which benefit your heart, muscles, and red blood cells. Crabs have no backbone and walk, swim, and even climb using their ten hinged legs. Interestingly, if a claw or leg is lost, it can grow back for survival.

Lobster

Lobsters are bottom dwellers found from the shore to the deep sea, on rocky, sandy, or muddy seabeds. Lobster has two powerful crusher and ripper claws with a hard shell that can shed its old shell and grow a new one in a process called molting. Lobsters have a long life expectancy, living for up to 100 years. They are orange, green, purple, and blue, naturally born with blue blood, but they turn red when cooked. Lobsters are carnivores that feed on fish, snails, clams, and other small animals. This diet gives us beneficial minerals like zinc, copper, protein, omega-3, and vitamin B. Although lobsters are higher in cholesterol, they provide nutrients essential for building and repairing body tissues, energy, and immune support, as well as brain function.

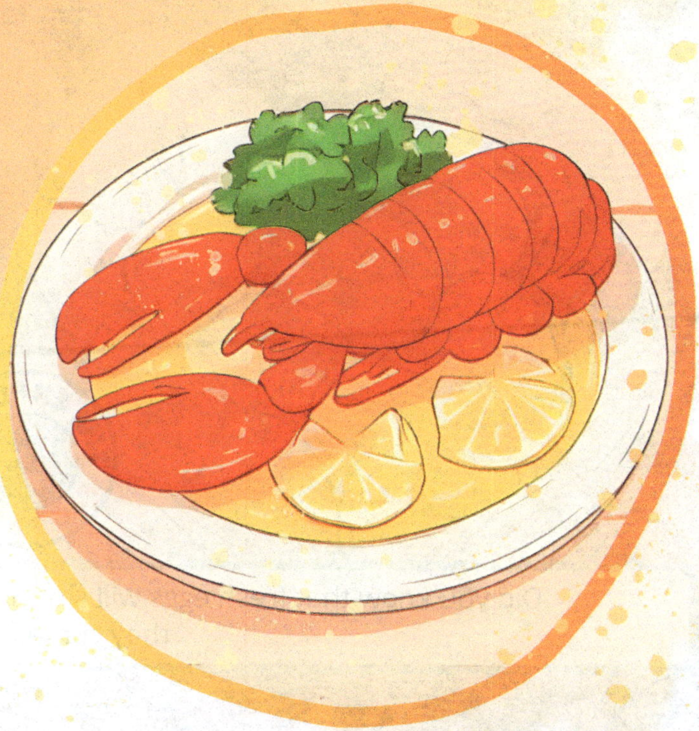

14. Eggs

Eggs are naturally protected by a sturdy shell and an ovoid shape that helps distribute pressure evenly, making them resistant to impacts and less likely to roll in a straight line. Edible eggs come from a wide range of animals, found on farms, coastlines, wetlands, and rivers. While chicken eggs are the most common, other edible varieties include duck, quail, goose, and fish eggs. Nutritionally, eggs are complete proteins, containing all nine essential amino acids needed for cell repair, growth, muscle function, memory, and energy. Eggs are also rich in vitamins A, B12, and D, as well as healthy fats that support brain and body health. Due to their high nutritional value and simple preparation, eggs can be enjoyed in many ways, including boiling, scrambling, poaching, and baking, across a wide range of recipes. In ancient Egypt, Persia, Greece, and Rome, the egg was a powerful symbol of fertility, new life, and rebirth, and eggs were often dyed and exchanged as part of spring festivals.

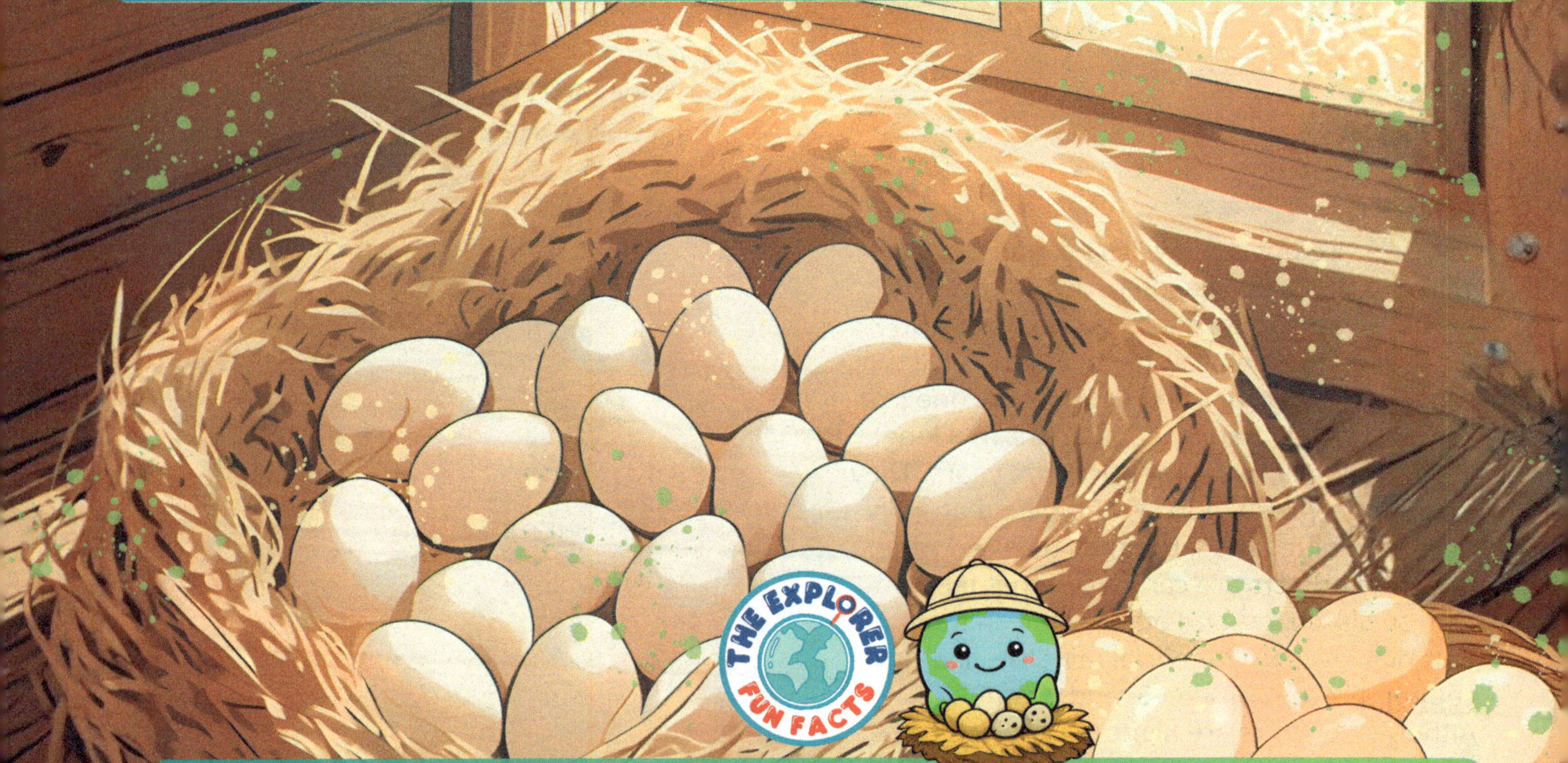

Did you know that fresh eggs will sink, but if they float, they're older because they contain more air.

Chicken Egg

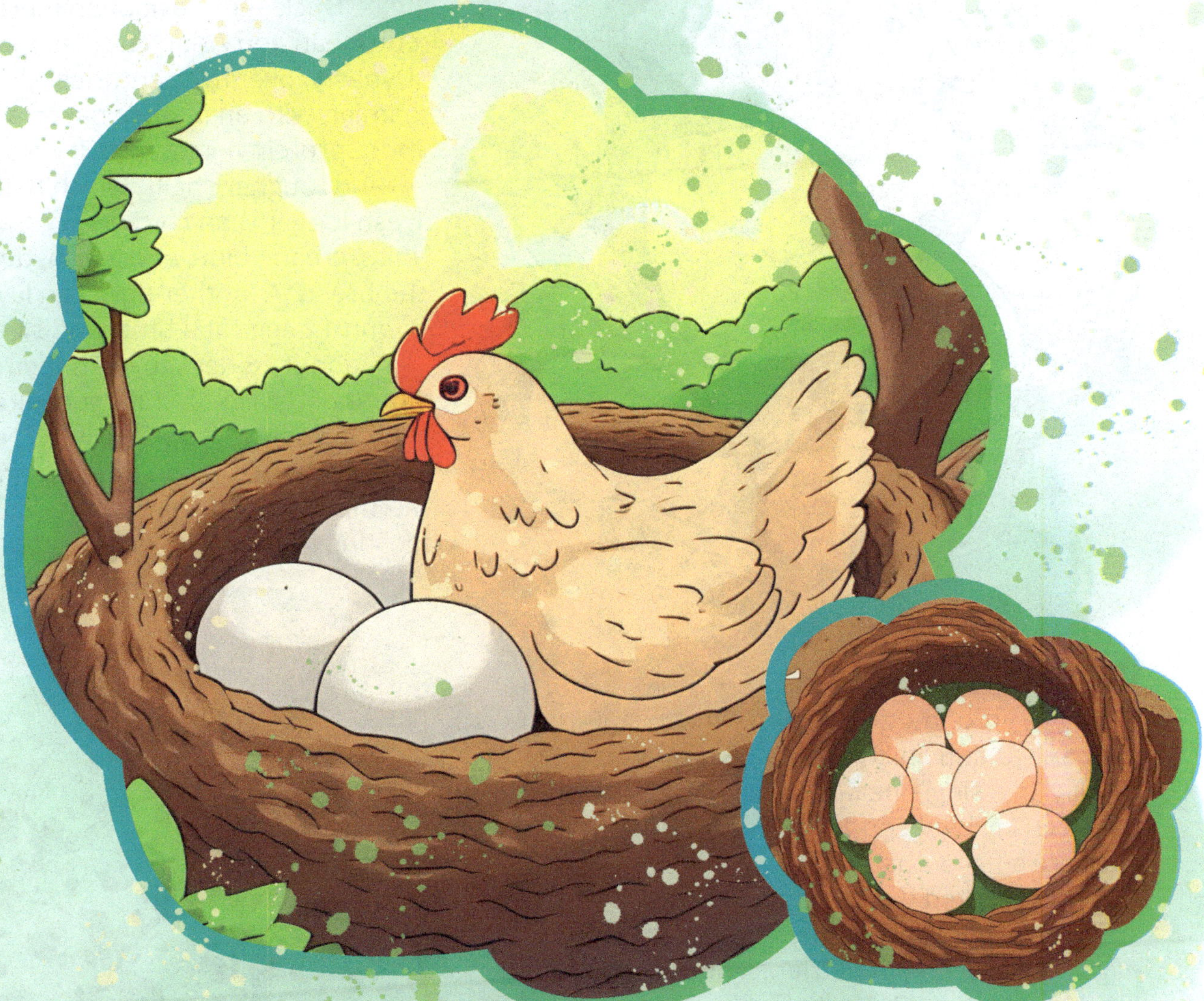

Chicken eggs are typically laid by the female birds called hens. Though a hen can produce more than 250 eggs annually, each egg takes roughly a day to produce. Chicken eggs can be white, brown, blue, or green depending on the breed, but the color doesn't change the flavor or nutritional value. They are a standard ingredient in many kitchens, rich in protein, healthy fats, vitamin D, and choline, which are essential for a healthy brain and help absorb vitamin E from vegetables. Eggs are easy to cook and great in any meal, providing lasting energy and fullness. The word "yolk" is derived from an Old English word meaning "yellow". The yolk is the more nutritious part of the egg, while egg whites offer low-calorie and fat-free protein ideal for restricted diets.

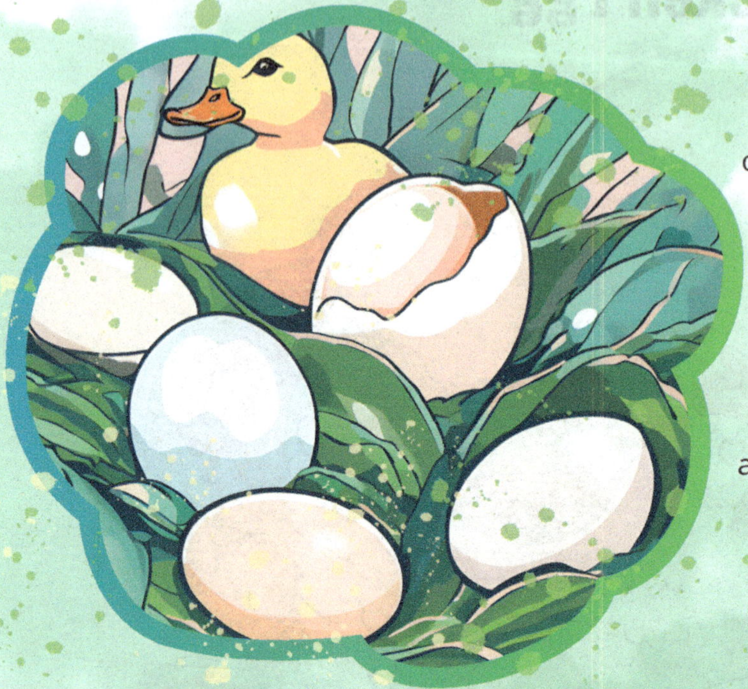

Duck Egg

Duck eggs have been more popular in European and Asian cuisines since the Ming Dynasty, over five centuries ago. The yolk is creamier, with an intense flavor, and contains more protein and fat. Duck eggs have larger and tougher shells, which help them stay fresh longer than chicken eggs, and come in white, cream, blue, and green, depending on the breed. A mother duck can lay between 5 and 12 eggs at a time, and sit on them for about 28 days to keep them warm. The amount of daylight a duck gets directly affects how many eggs she will lay. Nutritionally, duck eggs are rich in protein, omega-3, and vitamins, making them a fantastic choice for boosting brain health and promoting glowing skin and hair.

Quail Egg

Quail are ground-dwelling birds known for their speed and ability to escape predators quickly. In a single nesting season, female quail can lay between 12 to 16 eggs. These eggs are smaller than chicken eggs and can be easily spotted by their delicate, colorful, speckled shells. Despite their small size, quail eggs are packed with nutrients, including protein, iron, and B12, all of which contribute to healthy brain nerves and blood. It takes roughly three to four quail eggs to equal the nutrition of one chicken egg. Both quail meat and eggs are considered delicacies, especially popular in France, Poland, Italy, Mexico, and across Asian cuisines. Its creamy flavor is often enjoyed boiled, fried, poached, pickled, or in salads. They're also a great alternative for those with chicken egg allergies.

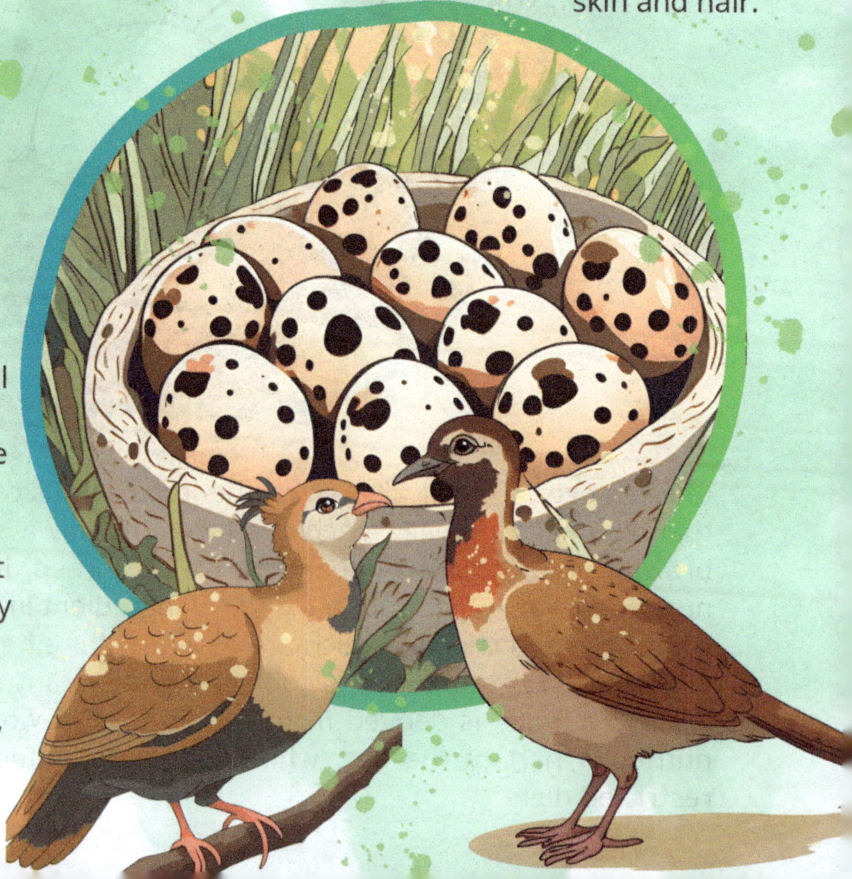

Caviar

Caviar comes from the salted eggs of sturgeon fish like Beluga, Osetra, and Sevruga. A single sturgeon can lay tens of thousands to even millions of eggs during one spawning season. Caviar is typically served on dark bread or blinis with cream or as a garnish on meals, known for its rich, buttery, and slightly briny flavor, with a smooth, melt-in-your-mouth texture, which has been highly prized since ancient times by the Greeks, Romans, and Russian royalty. Despite its size, caviar is highly nutritious, sought after for its richness in protein, omega-3 fatty acids, vitamins, and minerals. They support a healthy heart, reduce inflammation, aid brain function, and help prevent bone loss thanks to their high omega-3 content. Instead of chewing, caviar should be gently pressed against the roof of the mouth with the tongue to release its buttery flavor.

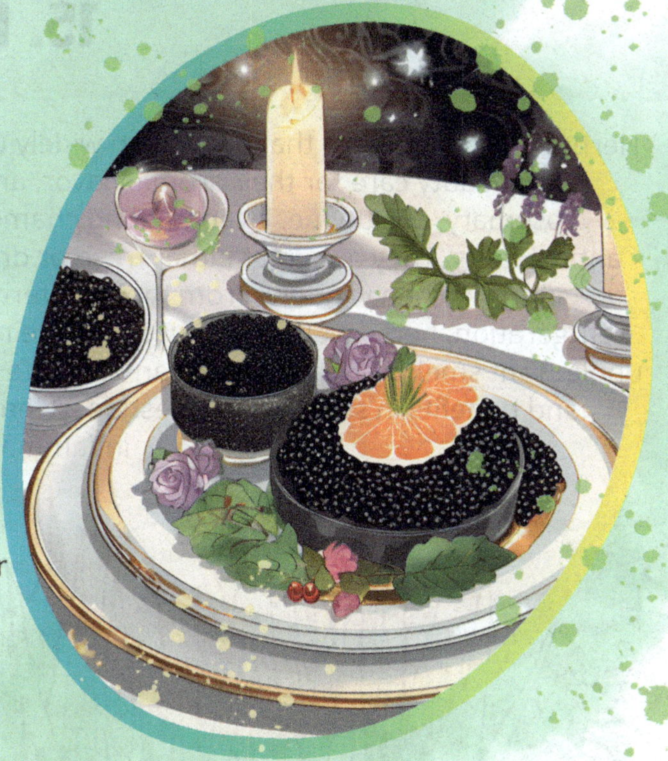

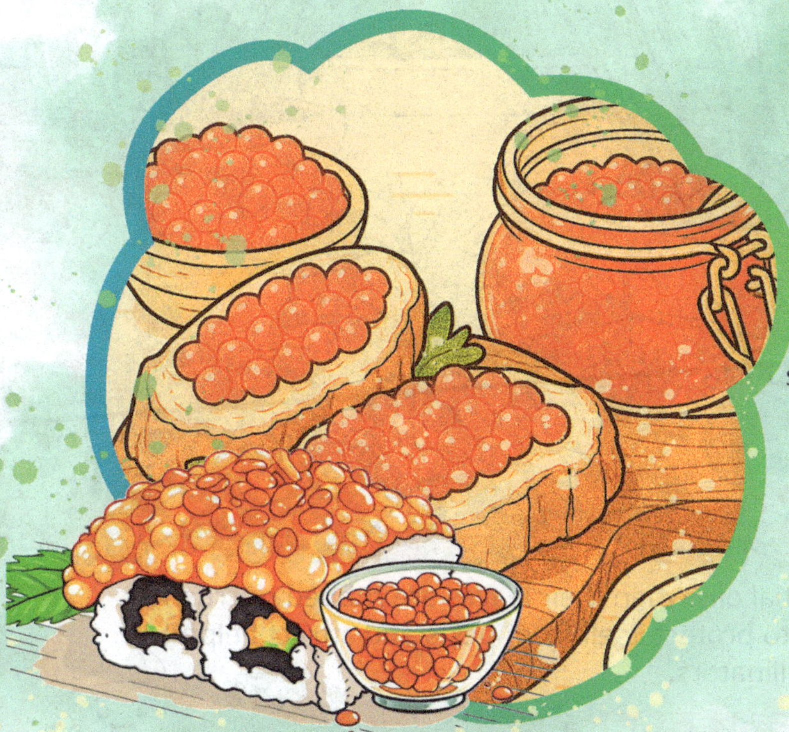

Roe

Roe are the eggs from almost any female fish, including trout, salmon, and even shellfish like scallops and shrimp. Some of the most common types include salmon roe (Ikura), flying fish roe (Tobiko), and capelin roe (Masago). Because it's less expensive, roe is more readily available and used in numerous cuisines, unlike caviar, which can only be sourced from the sturgeon species. Roe pops in mouth like tiny bubbles is often used as a colorful garnish for sushi, in appetizers, or as an ingredient in sauces and spreads. These tiny eggs are rich in healthy fats, protein, vitamins, selenium, minerals, and amino acids that enhance brain, body function, and immunity. The downside of roe is its high cholesterol and sodium content, a factor to consider for those on a health-conscious diet.

15. Herbs

Herbs are edible plants that have been widely used for centuries in cooking, medicine, rituals, and even beauty care for their aroma, flavor, and healing powers. Herbs such as basil, parsley, rosemary, dill, thyme, lavender, and chamomile are full of vitamins A, C, and K, as well as antioxidants. They are great either fresh or dried and easily grow in gardens, forests, fields, and sunny kitchen windows from the Mediterranean hills to tropical regions. Before modern refrigeration, herbs weren't just used for their flavor but also helped preserve meat and masked unpleasant smells. Just a sprinkle can bring life to any meal. Today, it is still used for its advantages and benefits in supporting digestion, strengthening immunity, and providing natural anti-inflammatory benefits.

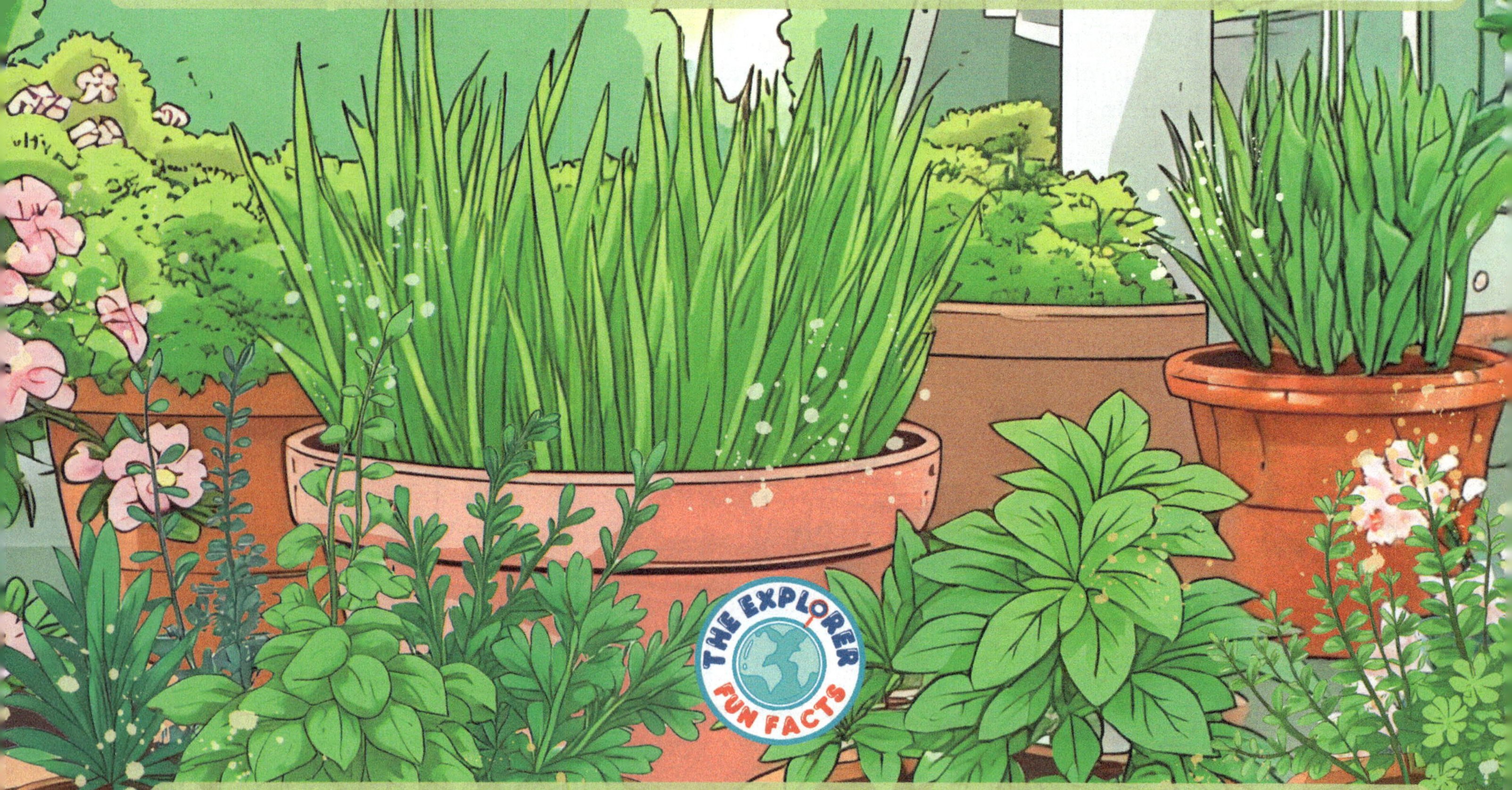

Many herbs release their scents and essential oils when their leaves are rubbed or crushed. It is part of the plant's survival strategy to protect itself from pests and attract helpful pollinators.

Basil

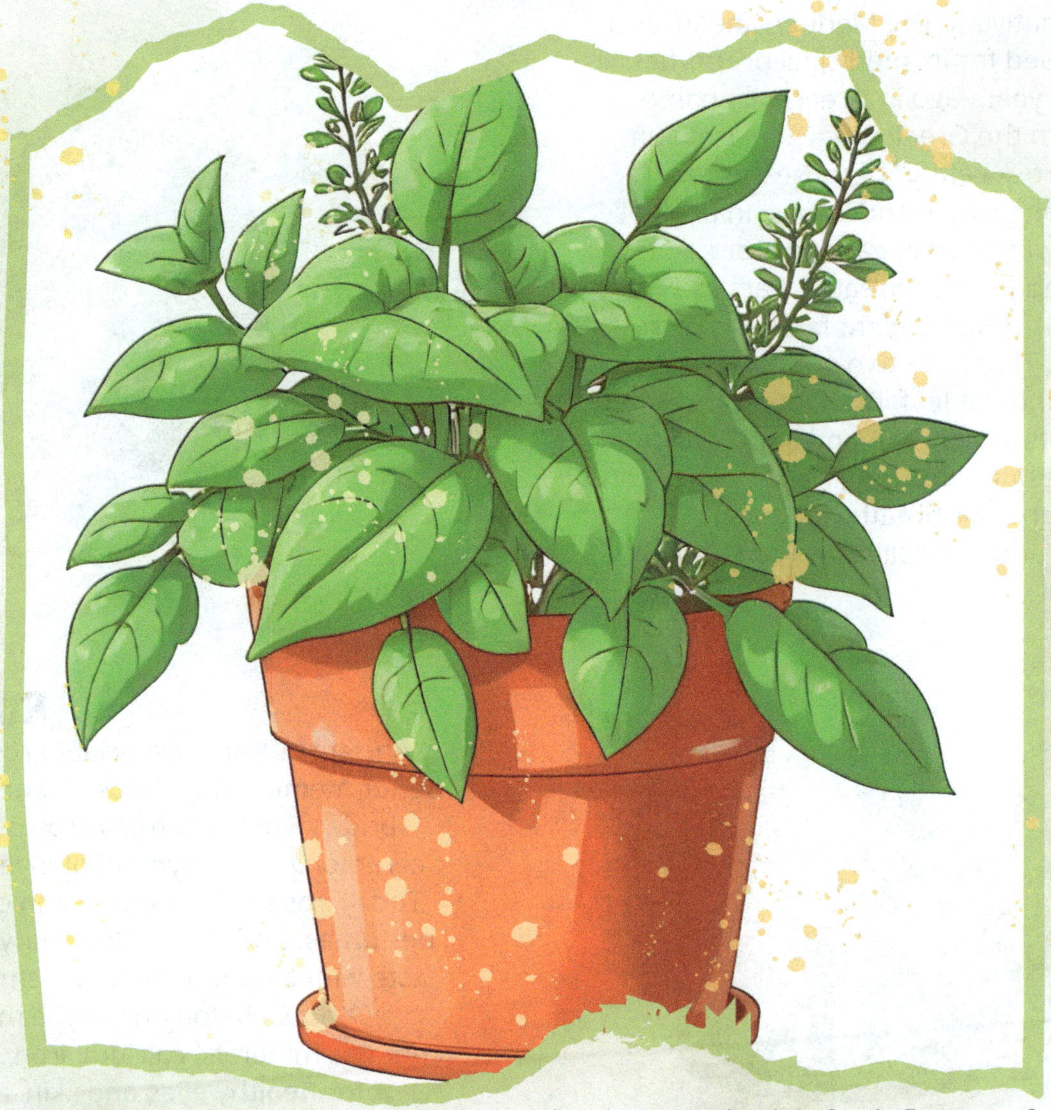

Basil is known for its lovely aroma and green color, bringing both a fresh flavor to food and health advantages. They thrive in warmer Mediterranean and parts of Asia regions with rich garden soil that are home to bees and butterflies. Italian cooking frequently uses basil to add a unique sweet and spicy flavor that is perfect for sauces and pesto. Basil is commonly added to pizza to infuse the flavor and appearance of a bright taste and vibrant green color. It is full of vitamins A, K, and C, as well as calcium and antioxidants that support the immune system. Chickens raised near basil plants often lay more vibrant eggs, thanks to the nutrients in their diet. In ancient times, basil was used for healing and in royal rituals. Basil can boost mood and naturally repel flies and mosquitoes.

Parsley

Parsley is native to the Mediterranean, and was first used for its medicinal properties over 2,000 years ago in Greece. Its name comes from the Greek word petroselinum, meaning "rock celery" because it often grows among rocky landscapes. In ancient Greece, it was used in garlands for game winners and funeral wreaths. Parsley belongs to the same plant family as carrots and celery. There are two popular types: curly leaf and flat leaf. Both types are rich in antioxidants, vitamins A and C, potassium, and magnesium. Chewing fresh parsley can help freshen your breath, and even butterflies and caterpillars enjoy snacking on it.

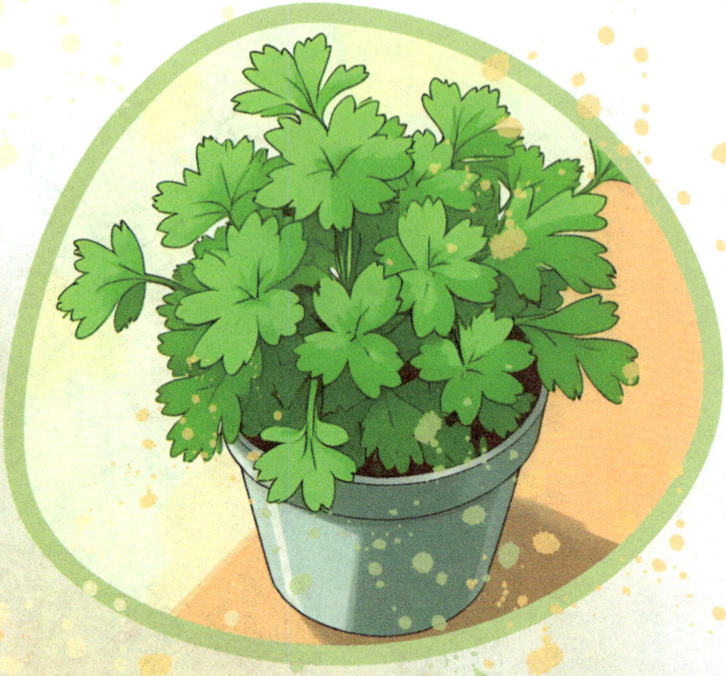

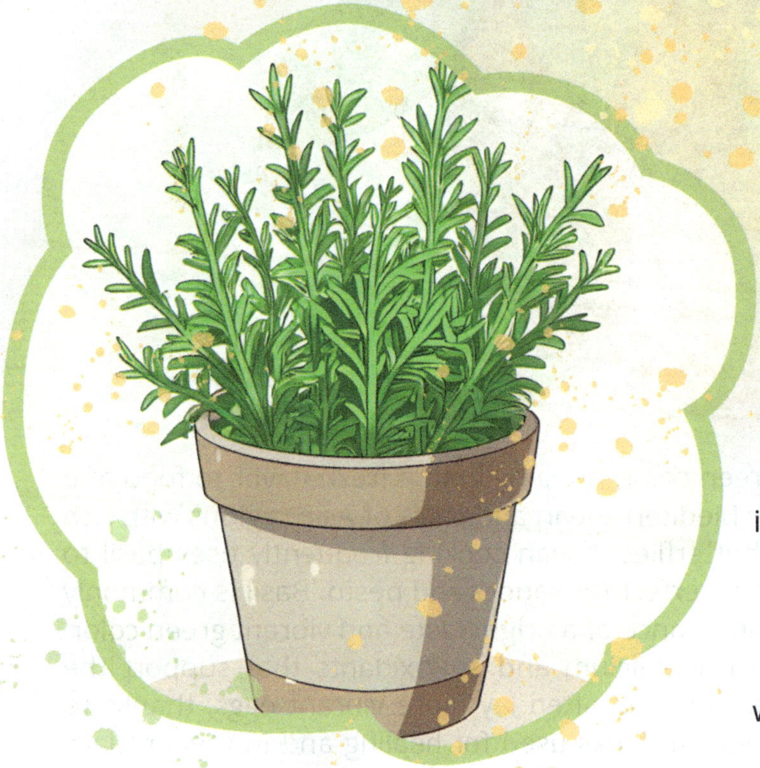

Rosemary

Ancient cultures associated rosemary with better memory and focus. In ancient Greece, brides wore rosemary crowns in wedding ceremonies as a symbol of love and loyalty. Today, rosemary is popular in cooking, oils, perfumes, and soaps. Rosemary has a bitter taste with a unique blend of lemon and pine notes belonging to the mint family. It contains minerals, calcium, iron, and vitamin A for healthy eyes and skin, and is rich in antioxidants that may help reduce anxiety, improve focus, and fight off sicknesses. When planted near vegetables, rosemary can naturally repel pests like mosquitoes, flies, snails, spiders, and slugs. The flowers are not only edible and flavorful, but they also help with pollination during springtime by bringing bees, bumblebees, and butterflies.

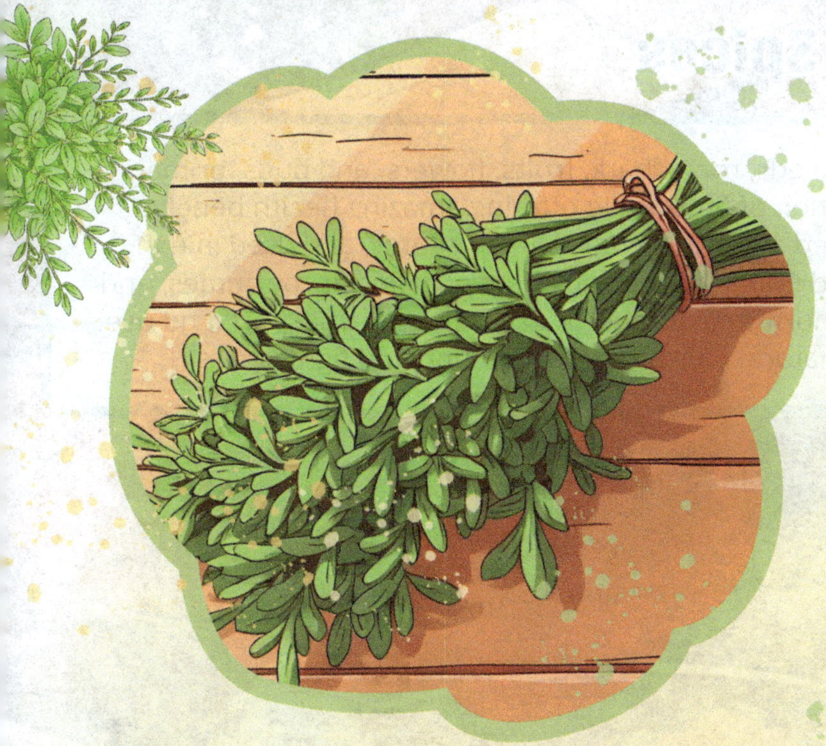

Thyme

The word "thyme" comes from the Greek word "thymos," which means bravery. To inspire bravery and fortitude, the ancient Greeks used thyme as incense in their temples. This tiny leafy plant is native to the Mediterranean and loved for its flavor, fragrance, and healing properties. Thyme is great fresh or dried to enhance the flavor of vegetables, meats, soups, stews, and pasta dishes. Thyme is safe for animals, and its pretty blossoms attract bees, helping produce delicious honey. Thyme is packed with antioxidants, vitamins A, B, and C, and iron, copper, manganese, magnesium, and potassium to support the heart, brain, skin, and immune system.

Oregano

The Greeks and Romans associated oregano with love and happiness, and used it in medicine to cure indigestion, fever, and poisoning. Today, oregano is essential in Italian, Mediterranean, and Mexican cooking, adding a distinct flavor to pizzas, pastas, salads, and sauces. Oregano has a strong and earthy taste, with a minty scent that intensifies when dried, making it last longer compared to some other herbs. Its savory flavor pairs well with tomato-based dishes, garlic, and onions. Nutritionally, oregano is rich in antioxidants, vitamin K, fiber, and minerals that support immunity, blood health, and disease prevention. Oregano has significantly more antioxidants than blueberries, oranges, and apples. So, start sprinkling this power herb in your meals.

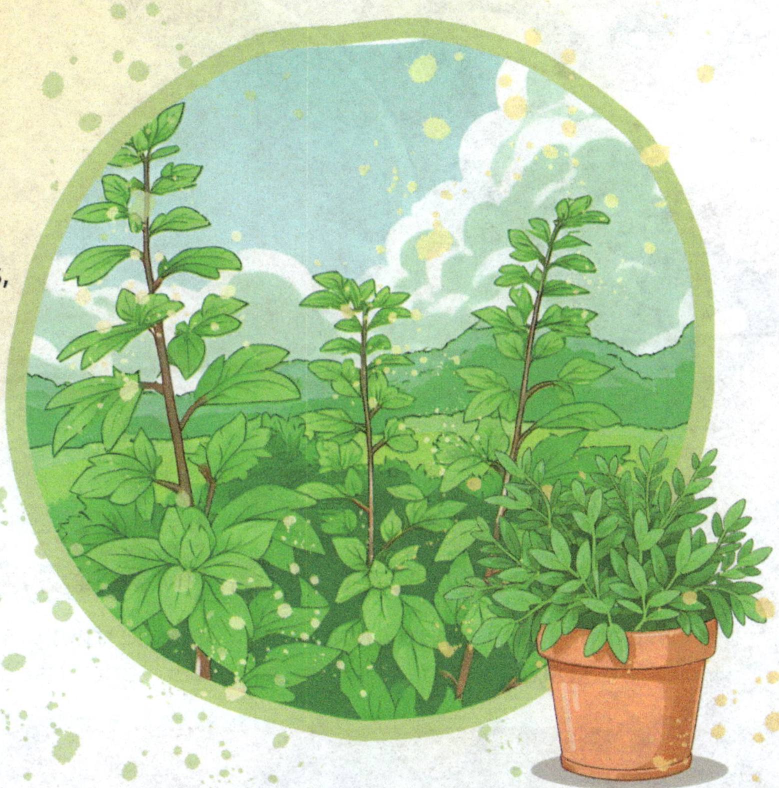

16. Spices

Spices are aromatic parts of plants, such as seeds, roots, bark, fruits, flowers, and buds, primarily used for flavor, aroma, color, and preservation of food while offering amazing health benefits. Spices have been valued for centuries, traded along ancient Silk Road routes, and used in early civilizations in Egypt, India, Mesopotamia, and China for religious rituals, medicine, perfumes, and cosmetics. Most spices are dried to remove moisture content for easy storage, transport, and use. It is full of antioxidants, minerals, and natural oils that help digestion and fight illness.

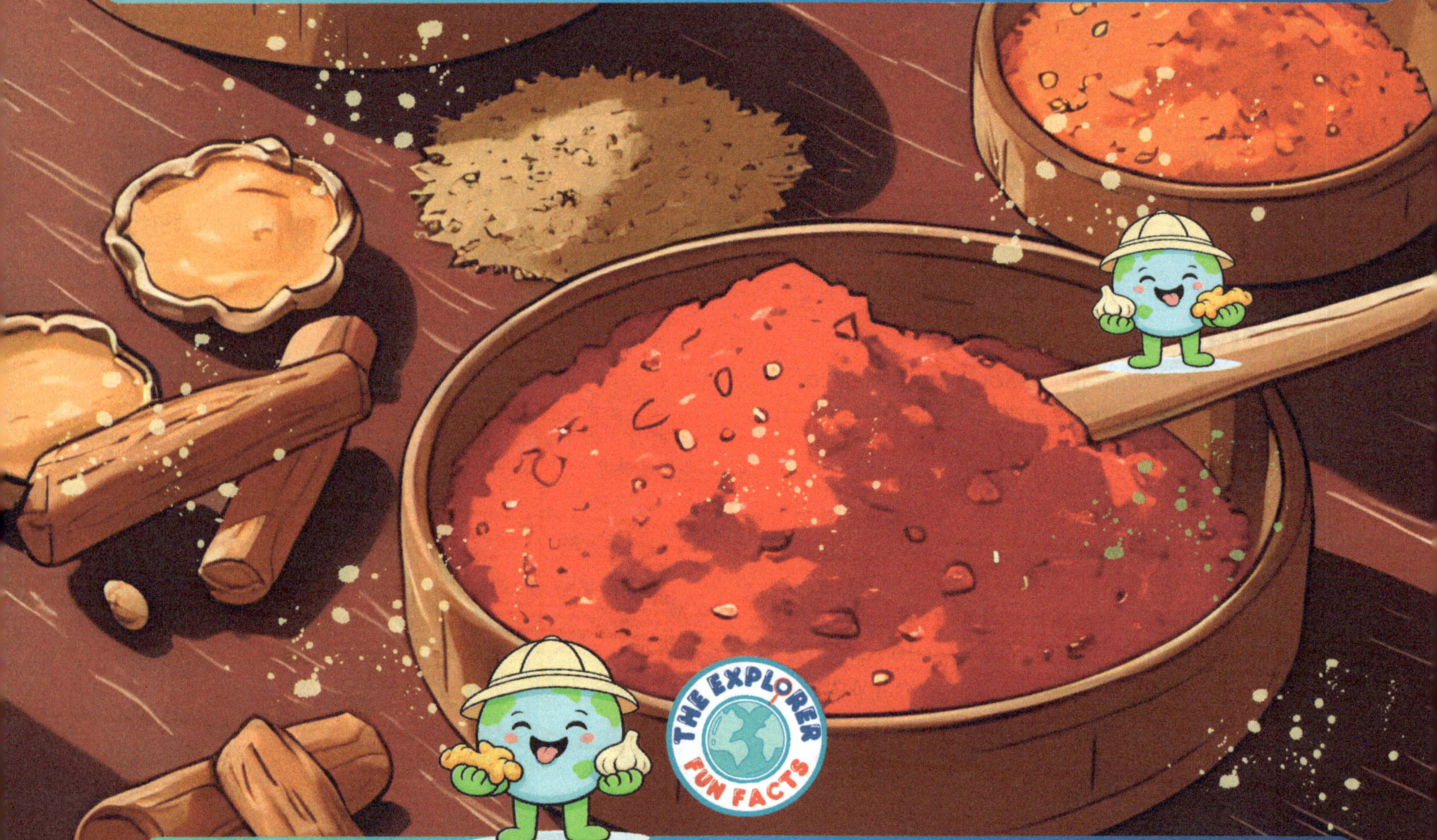

Some spices were once more valuable than gold and were used as a display of wealth and status. Pepper and nutmeg were once used as a form of currency and for ransom.

Garlic

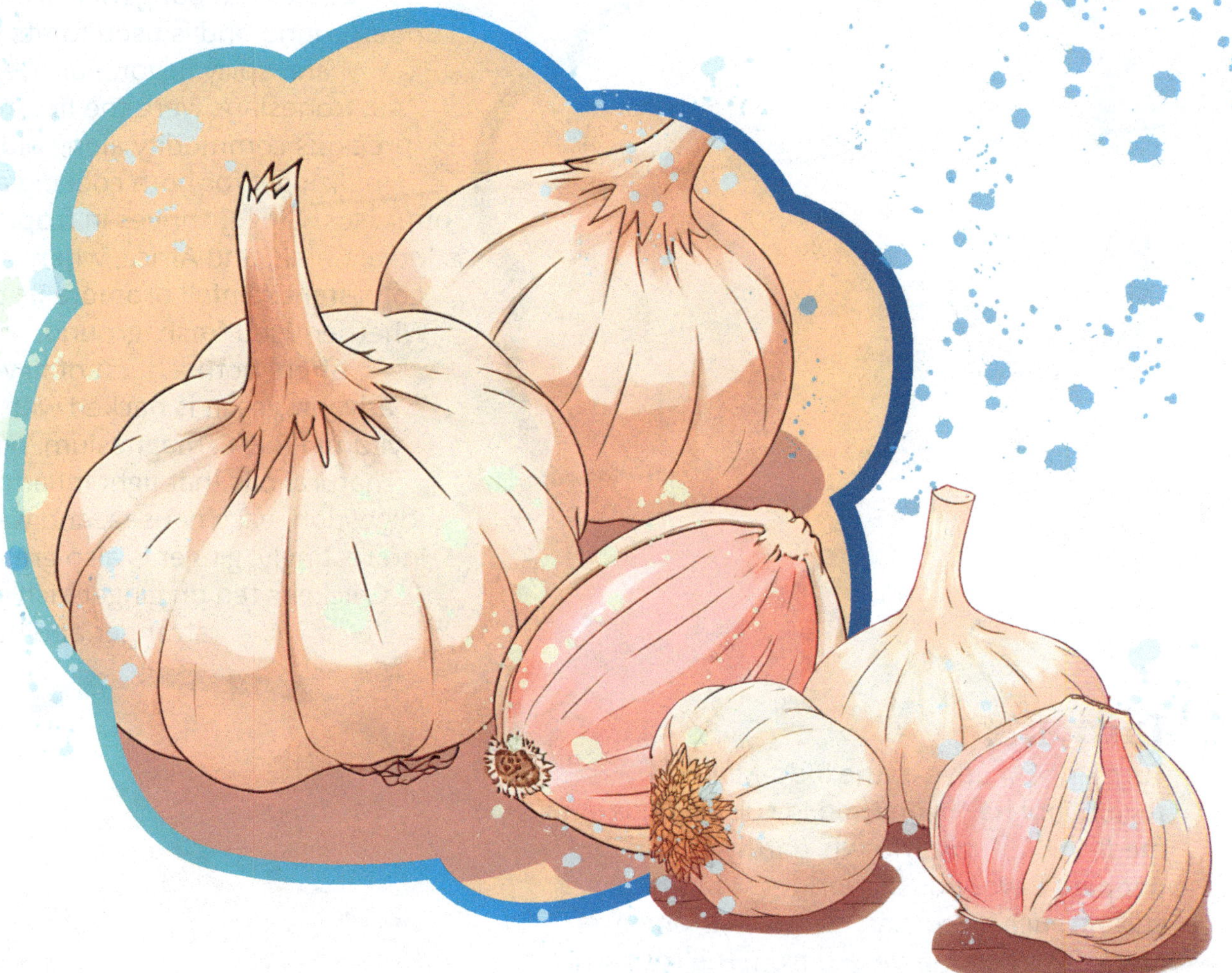

Although garlic is botanically a vegetable within the lily family, which includes onions, shallots, and leeks, garlic is commonly used as a spice. For centuries, garlic has been used in a variety of cooking, medicine, and even rituals. Since the Middle Ages, it's been believed to ward off vampires, monsters, and other evil spirits. Garlic is eaten raw or roasted for a pungent flavor, preserved or pickled for a milder and sweeter taste. Garlic is packed with nutrients like vitamins and minerals, including vitamin C, B6, and potassium, known to strengthen immunity, lower blood pressure, and reduce cholesterol. The Egyptians, Greeks, Romans, and Chinese all used garlic to treat many issues, including circulatory problems, parasites, digestive issues, and breathing troubles.

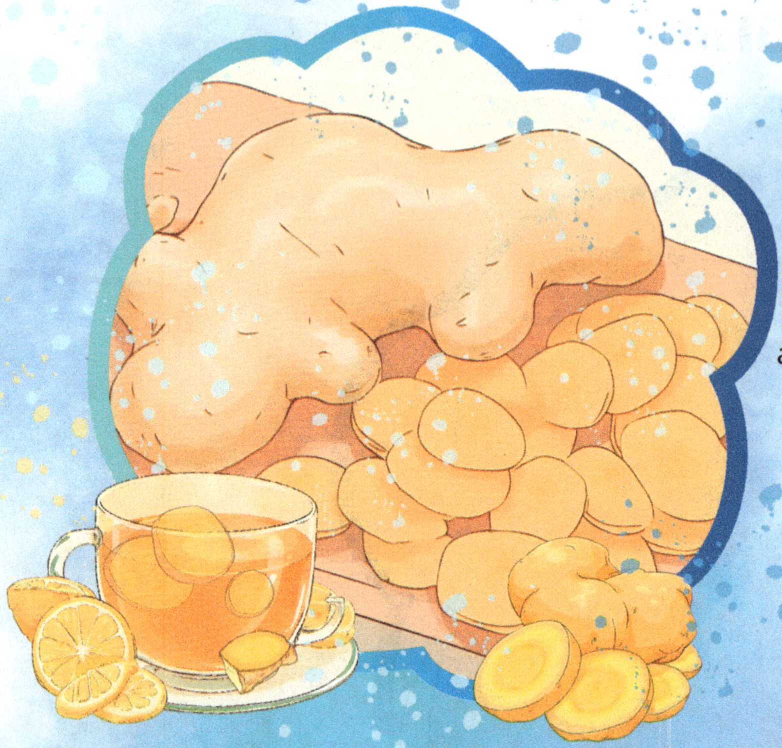

Ginger

Ginger is a pungent rhizome that grows underground and is used for its grassy aroma and spicy flavor. For over 5,000 years, Austronesians were the first to trade it as a precious commodity along old spice routes, utilizing it for both cooking and medicinal purposes. Ginger thrives in tropical areas such as India, China, and Africa, where fertile soil and consistent rainfall promote its development. Whether used fresh, ground, or dried, ginger offers both a burst of flavor and health advantages. It is packed with antioxidants, vitamin B & C, magnesium, potassium, and natural oils that fight inflammation, aid in digestion, ease nausea, and warm the body. Interestingly, ginger is also great for animals. Chickens fed on ginger-rich diets often lay stronger and healthier eggs.

Turmeric

Turmeric is native to the Indo-Malayan region and has been used in cuisine and medicine for centuries. Its earthy, bitter, and peppery flavor adds savoriness in Asian cuisine such as curries, soups, rice, and even tea. Turmeric is harvested from the root and is rich in vitamins A and B, with an active compound called curcumin that helps support the immune system and reduces inflammation. Curcumin is naturally fluorescent and can make water glow like liquid gold under a flashlight, turning the room into a glowing science lab. Its vibrant natural yellow color makes turmeric a popular choice for food coloring and fabric dyes. In nature, birds and chickens fed with turmeric can lay golden-yellow eggs.

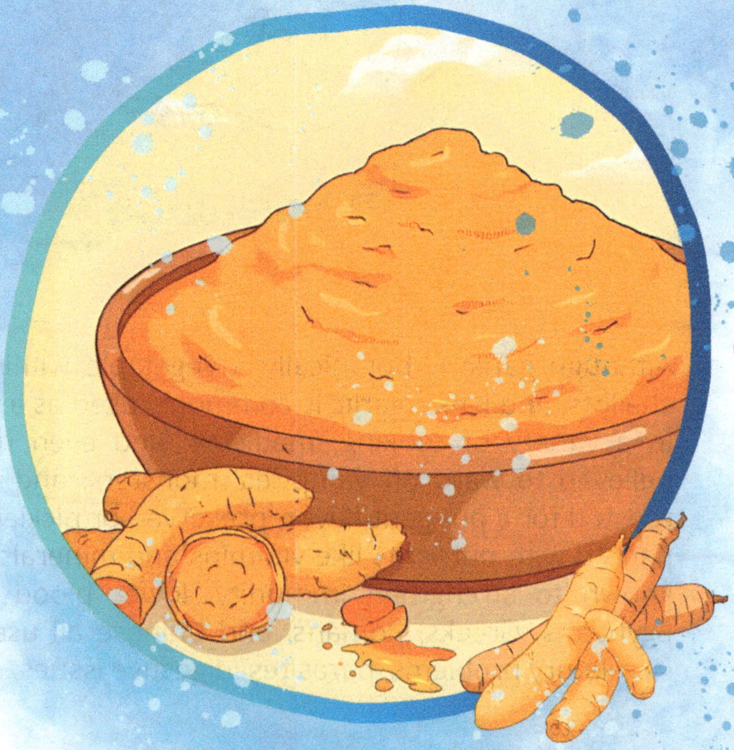

Pepper

Pepper is a spice that comes from various types of dried berries and fruits of plants such as black, white, and red peppercorns, cayenne, paprika, and chili peppers. The pepper flavor profile varies depending on the species and harvesting time. Spicy peppers add excitement, flavor, and satisfaction to more complex dishes in Asian, South American, Egyptian, and European cuisines. Peppers are full of fiber, antioxidants, vitamins A and C, which help improve digestion, metabolism, and inflammation. Uniquely, the heat and spicy flavor of the peppers come from capsaicin, a chemical compound that affects mammals, but animals like birds are immune to it.

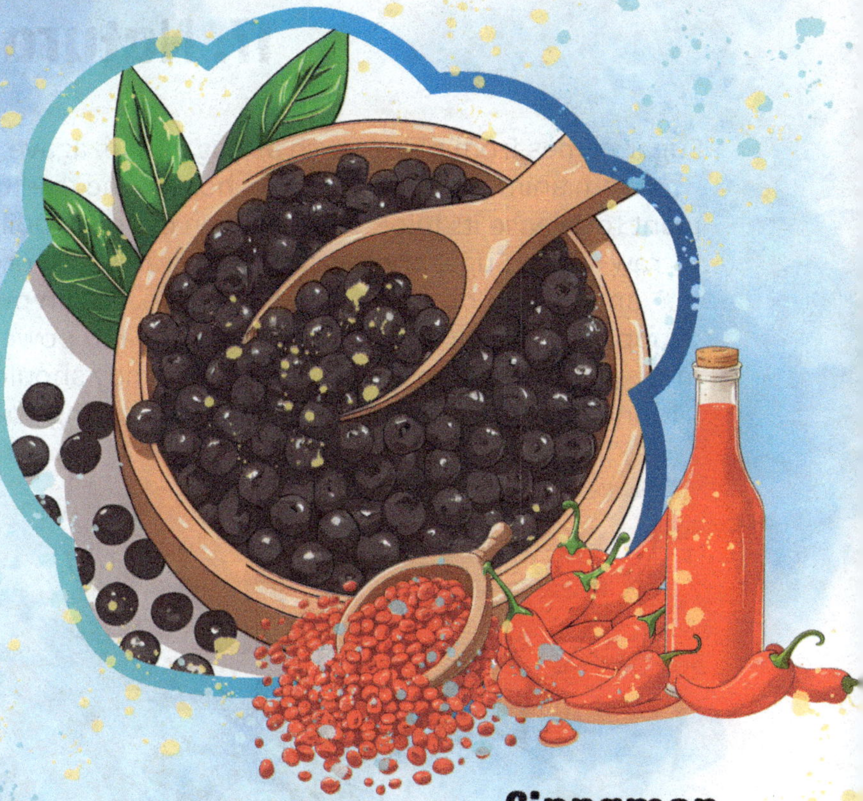

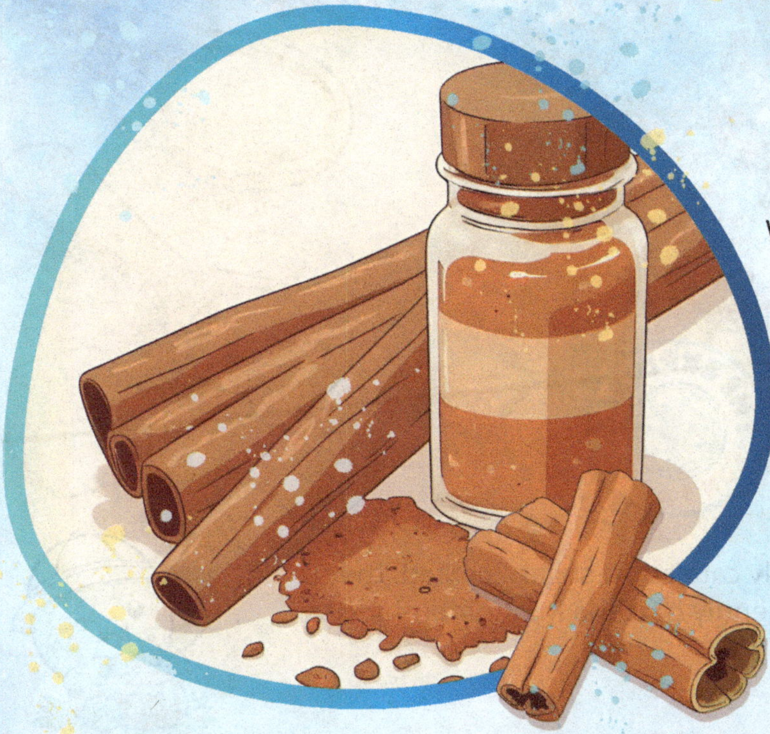

Cinnamon

Cinnamon is the dried bark harvested from a tree called True Cinnamon found in the tropical areas of Sri Lanka, India, and Southeast Asia. In ancient times, cinnamon was considered a luxury spice and a symbol of wealth, typically used in ceremonies, rituals, and medicine. In ancient Egypt, cinnamon was even used as a fragrance to preserve mummies. Nowadays, it's a favorite spice in baking, drinks, desserts, and fragrance for its spicy, citrusy, and sweet flavor. Cinnamon contains antioxidants, supports healthy digestion, balances blood sugar, fights off colds, boosts focus, and lifts your mood. In the West, it's a beloved ingredient during fall and winter holidays, adding flavor, scent, and festive cheer.

17. Natural Sugar

Sugar comes from plants such as sugarcane, agave, beets, corn, maple, coconut, and dates, as well as from animal sources, such as honey. The traditional extraction process involves crushing the plant to release its juice, which is then clarified, boiled to evaporate the water, and crystallized into raw sugar. Sugar contains carbohydrates that provide quick energy but contribute only small amounts of other essential nutrients. Within our body, sugar is broken down into glucose, supplying energy for our cells and brain and powering everything from clear thinking to physical movement. While foods like soda and candy should be enjoyed in moderation, the natural sugars found in whole foods are important for lasting energy, focus, memory, and overall brain health.

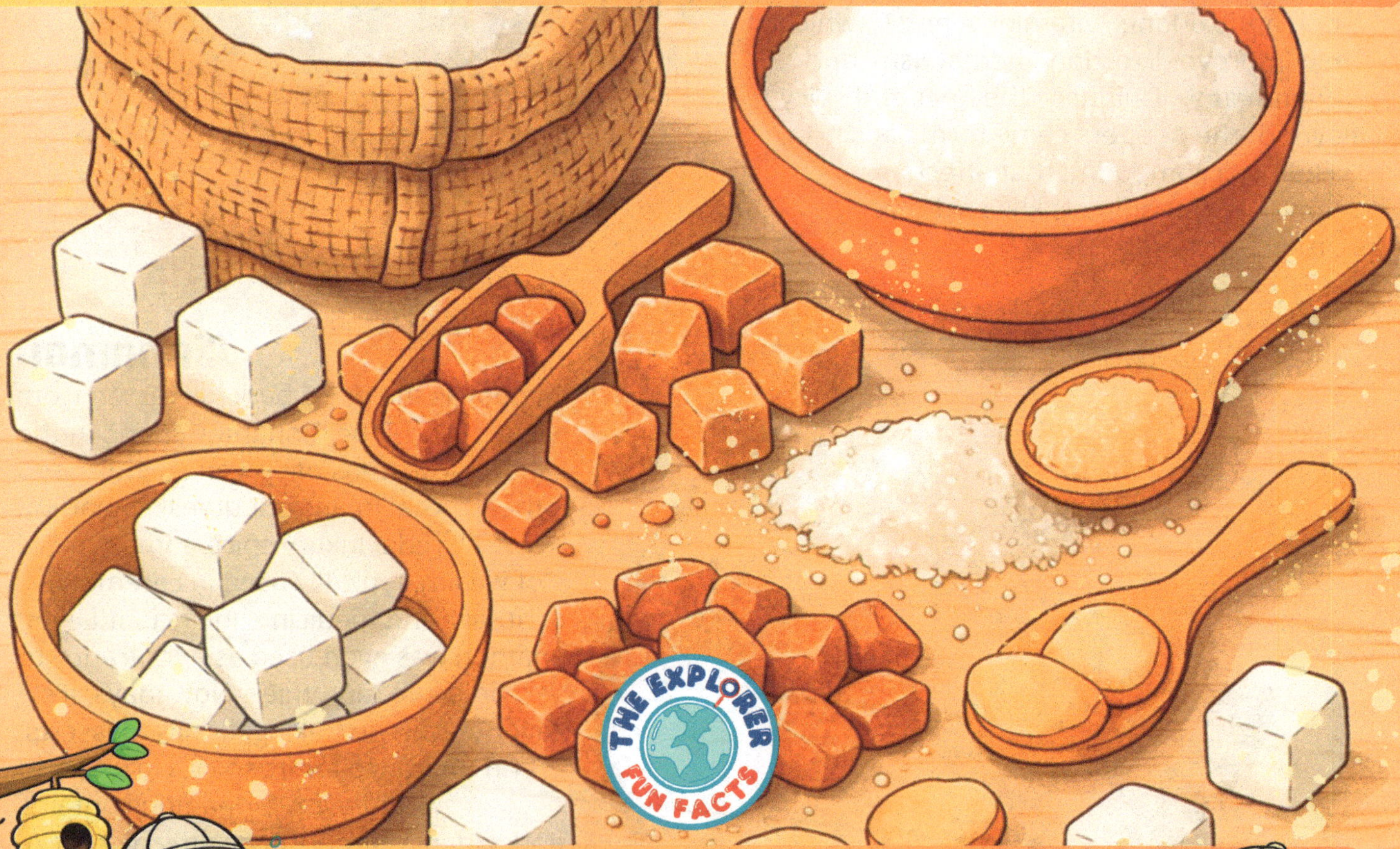

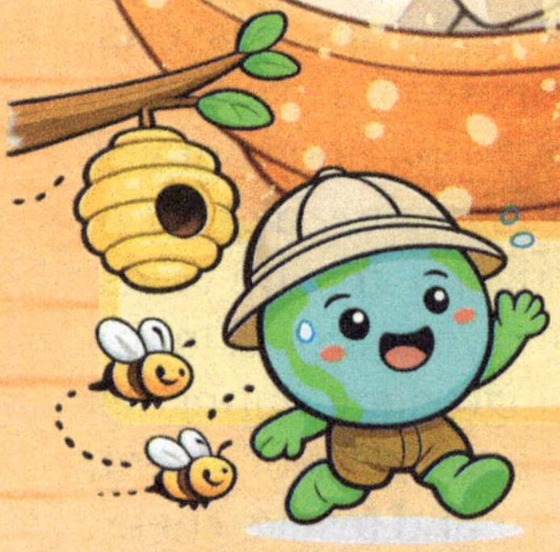

Cavities aren't directly caused by sugar. Instead, they're caused by unfriendly bacteria in our mouths.

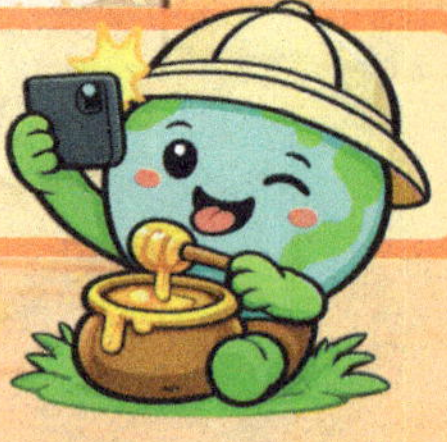

Sugarcane

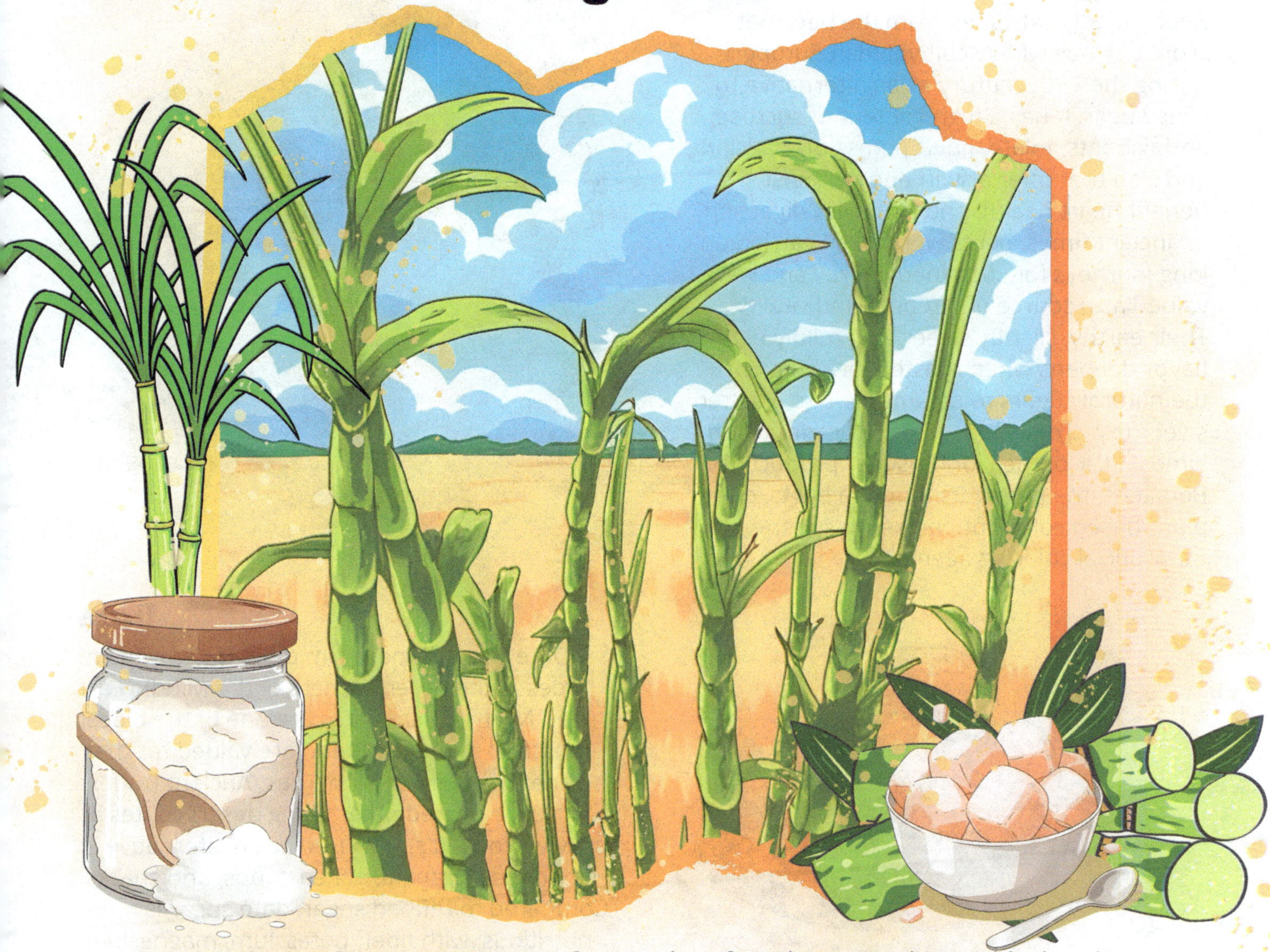

For hundreds of years, sugarcane, frequently referred to as "white gold," has been important in trade, culture, and medicine. I was first cultivated in New Guinea before spreading across Asia and the Middle East. Sugarcane is made by extracting the sugary juice, boiling it into a thick syrup, and evaporating it in a process called crystallization. It provides natural carbohydrates, small amounts of calcium, iron, and potassium, offering energy, electrolytes, and antioxidants. Consuming freshly squeezed sugarcane juice offers the most health benefits when done in small amounts. Even a little sugar can help sharpen your thoughts and lift your mood.

Beet

Beet sugar is extracted from the beetroot crop that was widely cultivated in Europe during the 18th century as an alternative to cane sugar. It has a high content of sucrose, antioxidants, folate, fiber, potassium, calcium, and iron that offer a swift energy boost, benefit heart health, and help with digestion. In ancient times, beets were often carried on long journeys for sustained energy and were valued as a source of strength and vitality. Their earthy, slightly sweet, and mildly bitter flavor deepens when roasted, bringing out the natural sugars to caramelize into a softer sweetness. Today, beet sugar contributes to almost 20% of the world's sugar production. Betalains, the pigments found in beets, offer plant-based color options, removing the need for artificial coloring agents.

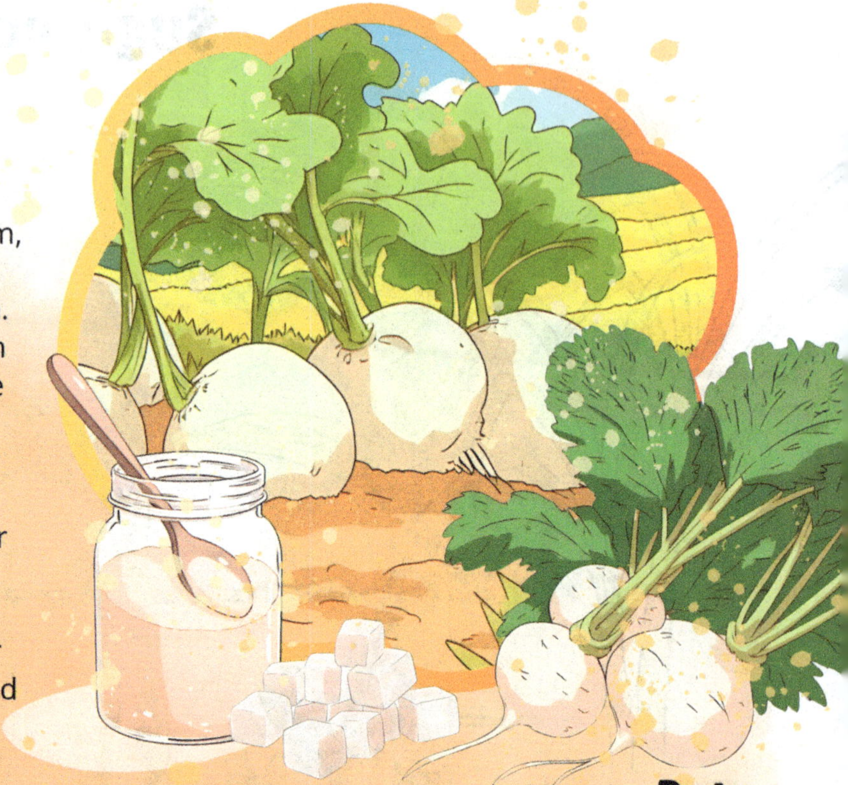

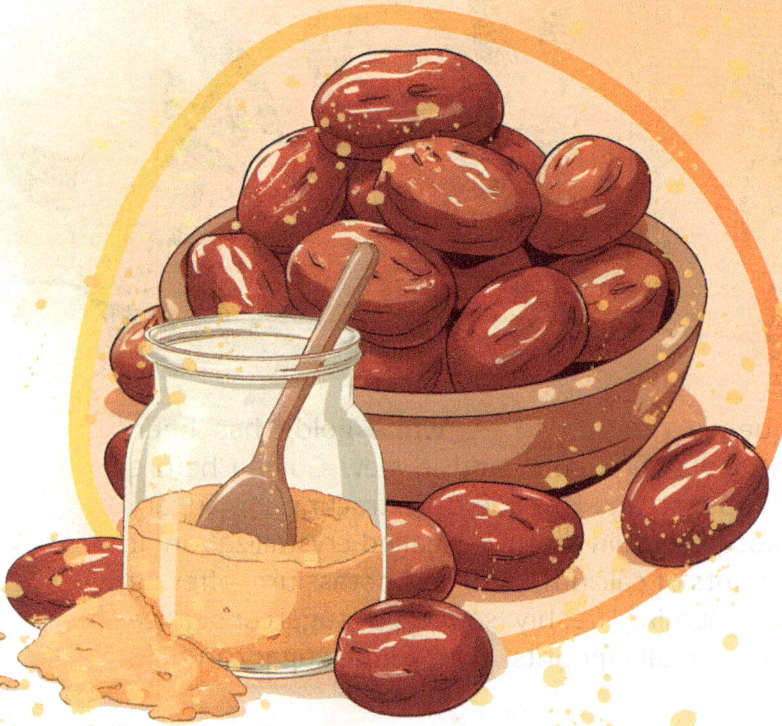

Date

Date sugar comes from dried dates of palm trees in the desert climate of the Middle East and North Africa. Dates are one of the oldest natural sweeteners and are valued for their energy-boosting properties. Ancient traders once carried dates along desert routes as survival food. It's now used as an alternative in smoothies, granola, baked goods, and snacks. Compared to refined sugar, date sugar is more nutritious, with fiber, potassium, magnesium, and antioxidants, which help your digestive system and fight inflammation. The sugar offers sustained energy, which the body can absorb slowly without causing a sudden drop. Because dates are a whole food, date sugar doesn't fully dissolve. Instead, it remains solid and settles at the bottom of beverages like coffee or tea.

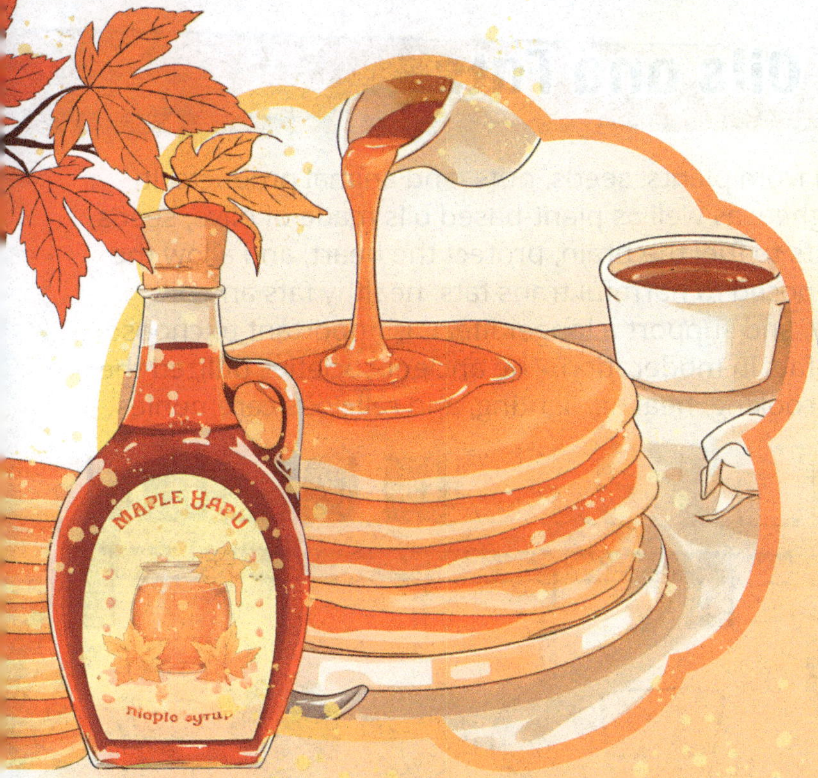

Maple

Maple syrup and maple sugar are natural sweeteners made from the sap of maple trees. It was first discovered by the Indigenous peoples of North America. Ever since, it has been a favorite not only as food but also as medicine. Maple sugar is often used to boost energy during long winters, preserve meat, and soothe coughs. It is rich in minerals such as manganese, zinc, potassium, and calcium, which help support bone strength, boost energy, fight inflammation, and protect cells. This sugar has a slightly lower glycemic index than refined sugar to avoid sharp blood sugar spikes. To get a gallon of maple syrup, you need to process about 50 gallons of sap. But the outcome is a rich, sugary, and caramelized flavor that satisfies cravings for sweets, especially on hot pancakes.

Honey

Honeybees gather nectar from flowers and store it in their stomachs. The evaporated moisture inside the hive causes the nectar to thicken, producing a viscous liquid called honey. Honey's flavor and color shift according to the floral sources bees visit, ranging from delicate and mild to robust and bold. Honey contains natural sugars like glucose and fructose, as well as trace amounts of antioxidants, enzymes, vitamins, and minerals. Incorporating honey into your diet in moderation is a flavorful and natural way to help maintain lasting energy and promote overall health. A single honeybee can create about one-twelfth of a teaspoon of honey in its lifetime, which requires visits to two million flowers to produce a single pound!

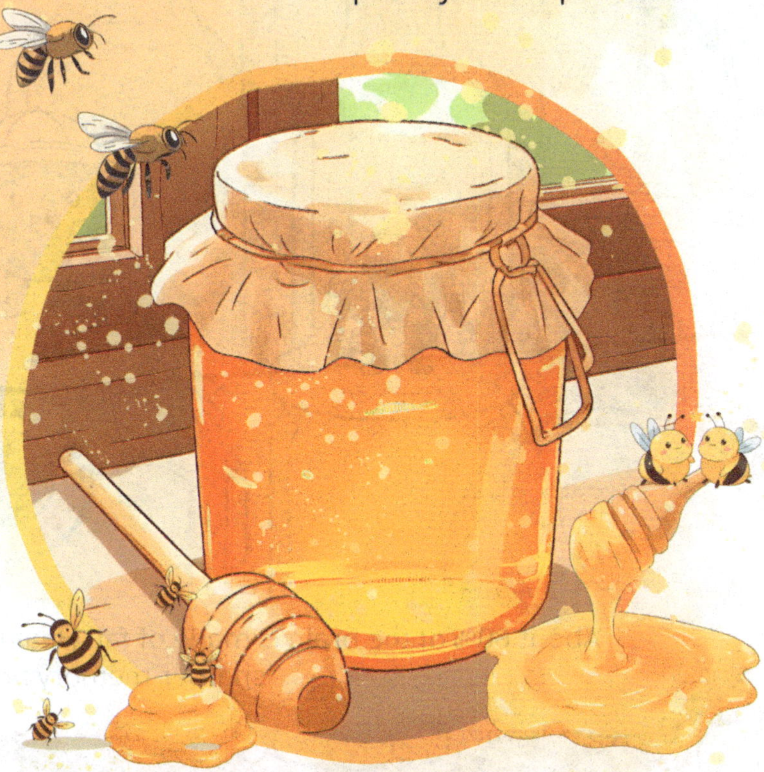

18. Healthy Oils and Fats

Healthy fats and oils are naturally sourced from plants, seeds, nuts, and animal products. It includes animal fats such as tallow, lard, and ghee, as well as plant-based oils made of olive, seeds, and coconut. Fats provide important nutrients to fuel the brain, protect the heart, and allow the body to absorb necessary vitamins. As opposed to harmful trans fats, healthy fats and oils contribute to a balanced diet, provide energy, and support a longer life. It is important to choose the kind and amount of fats and to consume fats in moderation. The ancient societies utilized the advantages of fats in various ways, including cooking, healing, lighting, and religious ceremonies.

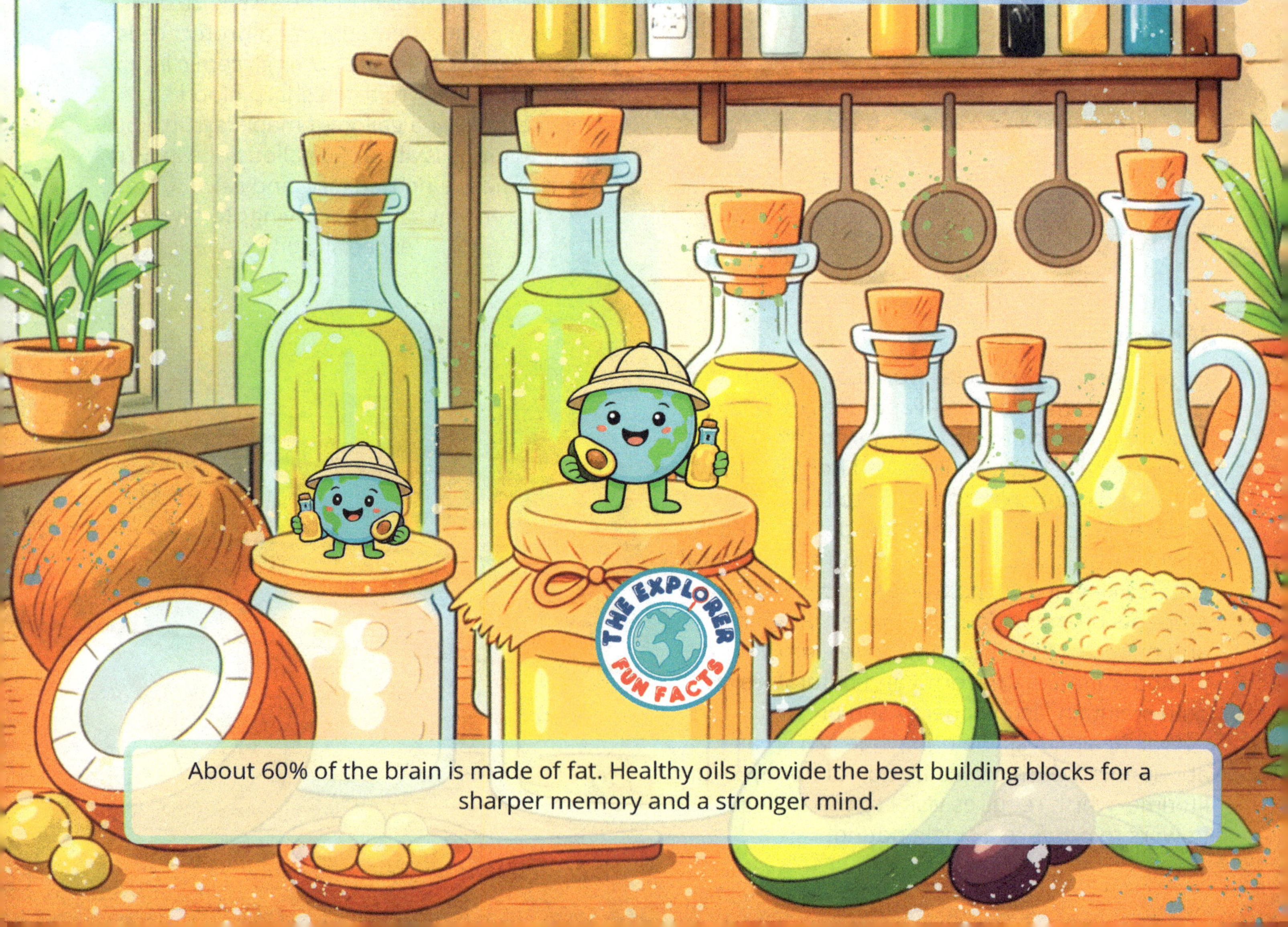

About 60% of the brain is made of fat. Healthy oils provide the best building blocks for a sharper memory and a stronger mind.

Olive Oil

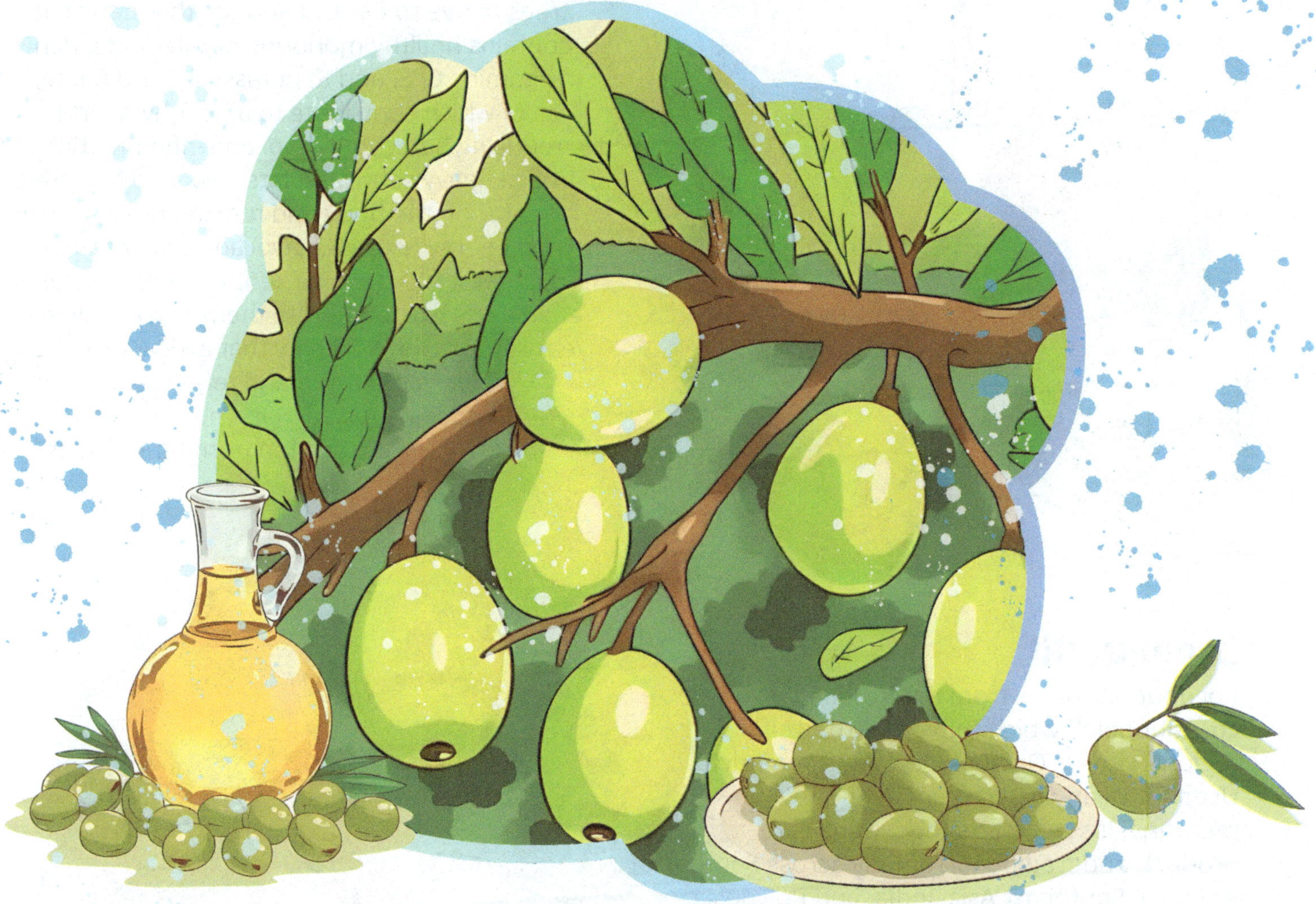

Olive oil comes from the olive tree native to the Mediterranean regions. It has been an important part of the region's culture, food, medicine, and rituals for thousands of years. In fact, olive branches were once used to crown Olympic champions, symbolizing strength, vitality, and growth. The oil is rich in healthy monounsaturated fats, antioxidants, and chemical compounds that give olive oil a nutty, fruity, bitter, and pungent flavor. It has medical properties that reduce inflammation, protect against heart disease, and prevent damage to your body's cells. Unlike other vegetable oils that require intense chemical and heat processing, extra-virgin olive oil is produced using a simple crushing and pressing method. Olive oil is technically a fruit juice. You are consuming the pure goodness of nutrient-rich fruits, a staple in the healthy Mediterranean diet.

Avocado

An avocado is a fruit that grows on evergreen trees native to Central and South America. It contains healthy monounsaturated fats, rich in vitamins C, E, and K, potassium, and folate, all of which contribute to a healthy heart by reducing bad cholesterol and inflammation. Unlike heavy saturated fats, avocado fats are lighter on the body and fuel the brain, skin, and energy levels. An avocado will not ripen until after it has been picked. This unique trait enables us to incorporate them into our diets year-round. Did you know that avocados have more potassium and fewer carbs than bananas and can help improve nutrient absorption from other foods?

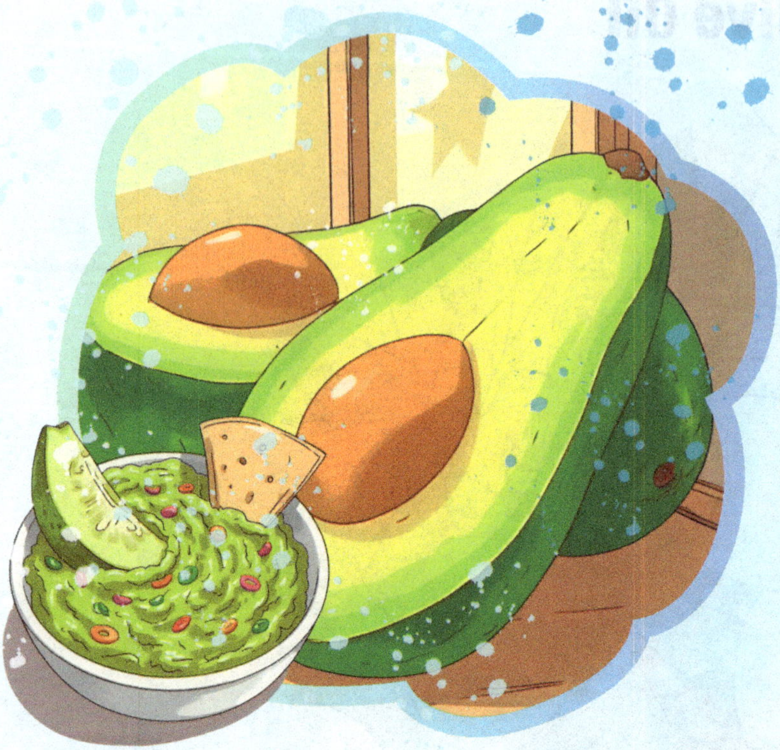

Coconut Oil

Coconut oil comes from the fruit of the coconut palm, which thrives in tropical regions of Asia, Oceania, and South America. Used for nearly 4,000 years in ancient medicine, it served as a food, body care product, and traditional remedy across South America, Southeast Asia, India, and Polynesia. Coconut oil has a nutty and sweet flavor, and it contains medium chain triglycerides (MCTs), which the body quickly converts into energy. These nutrients support healthy cholesterol levels, brain function, and provide quick energy. Though high in saturated fat, it's best enjoyed in moderation. Because of its low melting point, coconut oil works well as a natural alternative to butter.

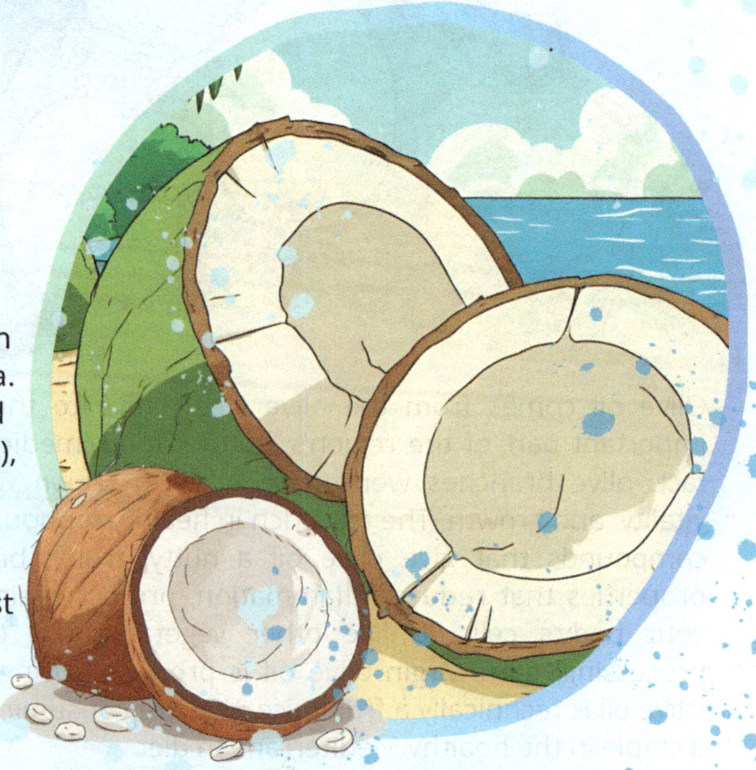

Fish Oil

Fish oil is primarily sourced from oily fish, such as salmon, cod, mackerel, and sardines, that live in cold ocean waters. The ancient Nordic people viewed it as precious liquid gold because it gave strength and helped them survive through the long and cold winters. The richness of Omega-3 fatty acids, including EPA and DHA, and vitamin D in fish oil is crucial for good brain health, decreasing inflammation, and safeguarding joints and skin. Fish oil has powerful anti-inflammatory properties that can help ease arthritis conditions and even lower the risk of heart disease and high blood pressure. Our bodies cannot produce omega-3 fatty acids naturally. Therefore, including fish oil in our diet is like giving the body a daily tune-up for optimal wellness.

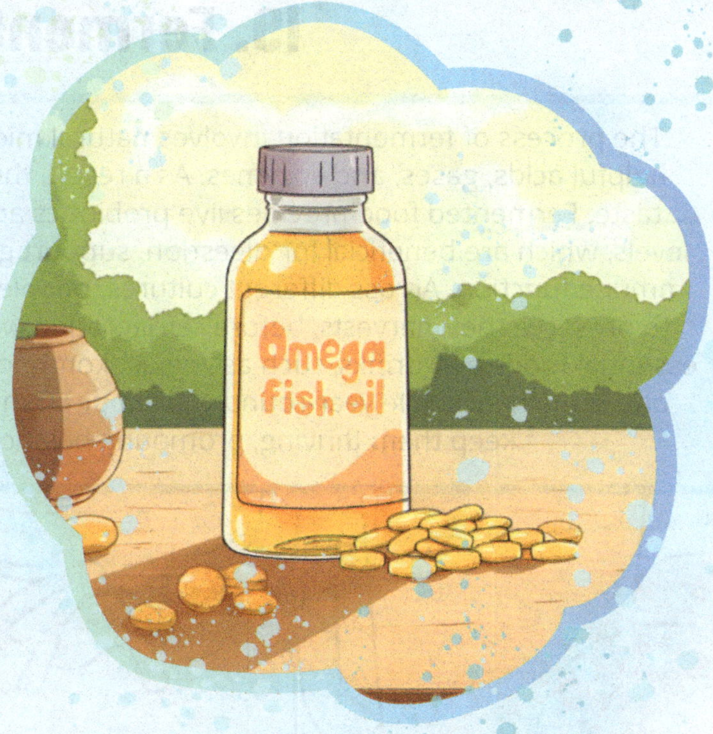

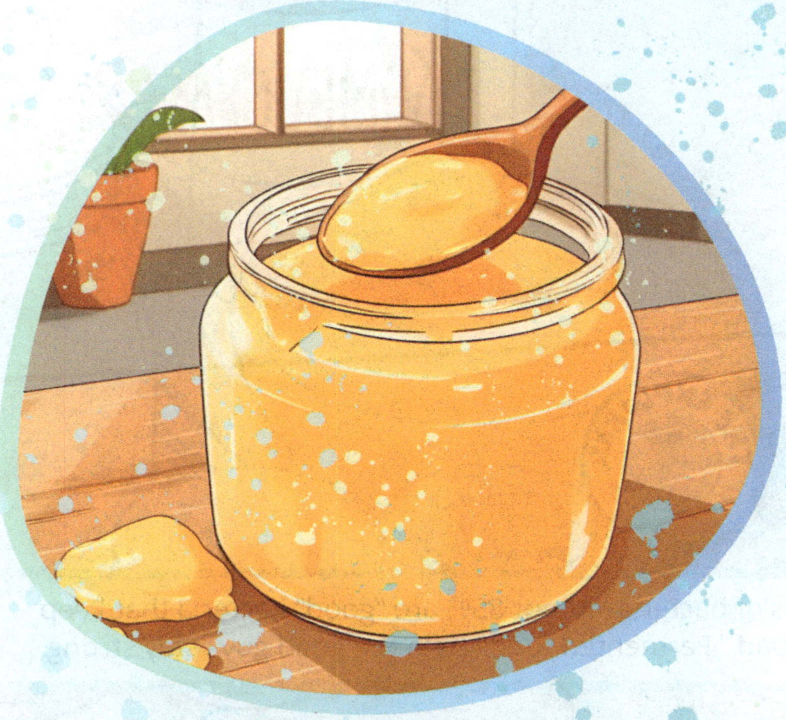

Ghee

Ghee is created by slowly heating butter to separate the solids, resulting in a transparent and golden fat with a nutty flavor, also known as clarified butter. Ghee is often used in Middle Eastern and Asian cultures for both culinary purposes and traditional medicine. For centuries, ghee has been a symbol of both purity and strength. Ghee contains vitamins A, D, and E, along with healthy fats, which promote good gut health, reduce inflammation, and aid digestion. This cooking oil is great because it can withstand high heat, so it won't degrade and become harmful.

19. Fermented Foods

The process of fermentation involves natural microorganisms that alter the food and generate helpful acids, gases, and enzymes. As a result, the method preserves the food and improves its taste. Fermented food provides live probiotics and increases vitamin, mineral, and antioxidant levels, which are beneficial for digestion, support gut health, reduce inflammation, and strengthen immune function. Across different cultures, people have used fermentation for thousands of years to preserve their harvests, before refrigeration was available. This process has provided us with essential foods and drinks, such as yogurt, kombucha, sauerkraut, and kimchi, that extend shelf life and remain available year-round. Since our gut hosts trillions of bacteria, fermented foods help keep them thriving, promoting balance, vitality, and smarter diet choices.

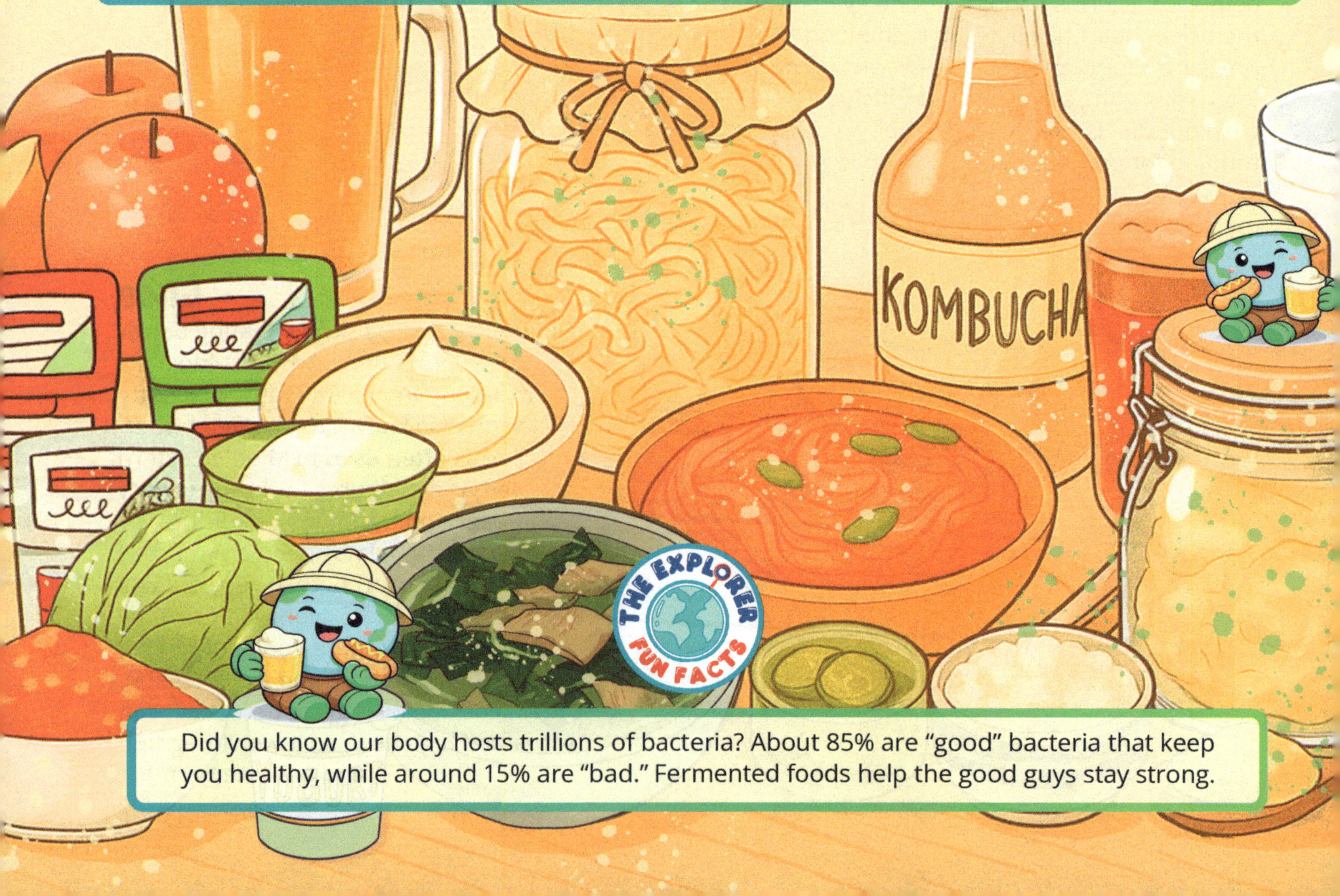

Did you know our body hosts trillions of bacteria? About 85% are “good” bacteria that keep you healthy, while around 15% are “bad.” Fermented foods help the good guys stay strong.

Sauerkraut

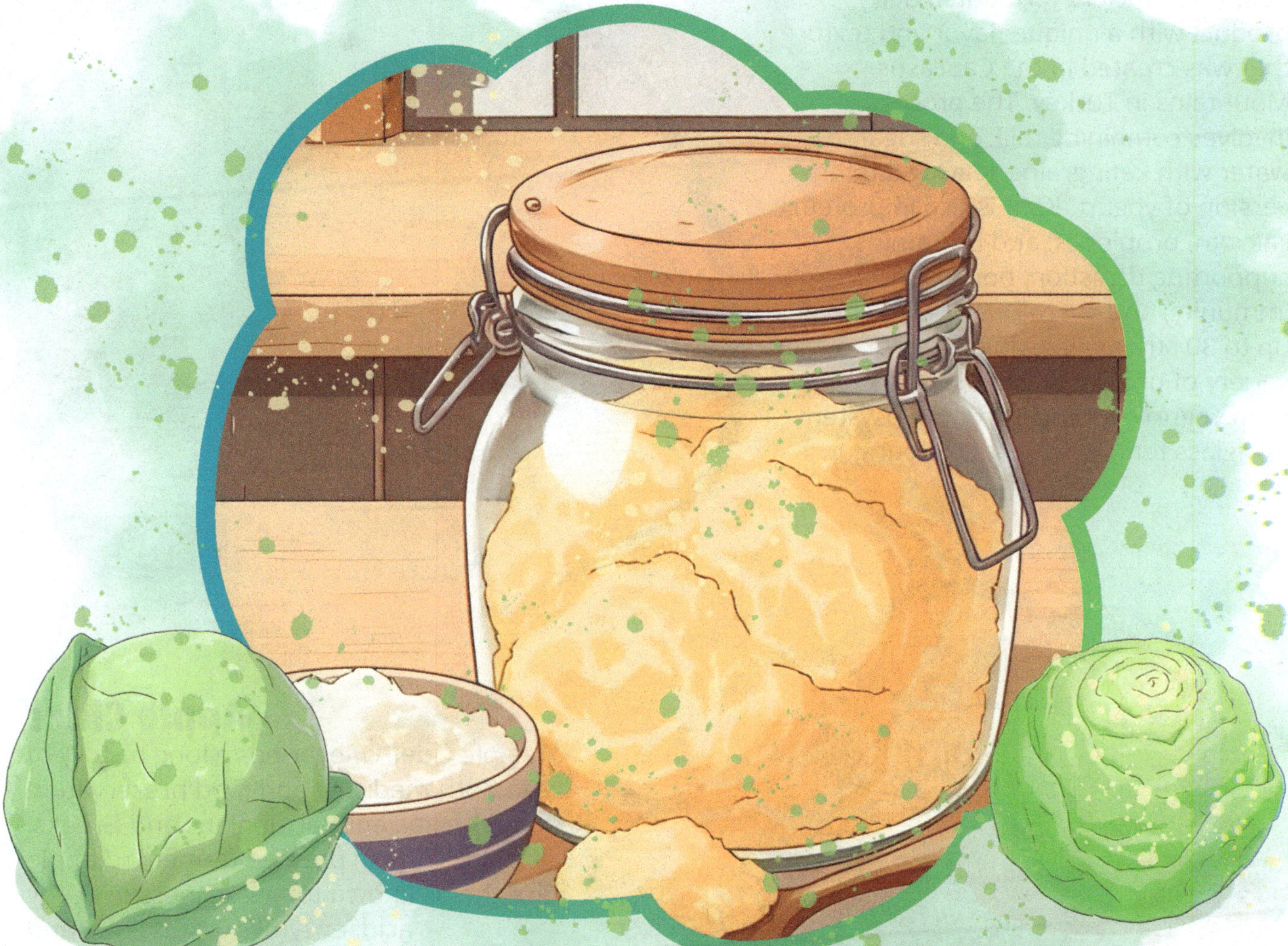

Sauerkraut, means "sour cabbage" in German, was first produced over 2,000 years ago during the construction of the Great Wall of China. It later gained popularity in Europe and became sailors' favorite food during long voyages to avoid scurvy. Sauerkraut is made by letting cabbage sit in its own juices for a while, to help good bacteria grow and give it a sour taste, providing probiotics, vitamin C, K, fiber, and minerals. The fermentation process preserves nutrients while introducing beneficial bacteria that support gut health and provide a natural boost to digestion and immunity. Adding sauerkraut to your diet can help balance cravings, as its tangy flavor satisfies the palate while nurturing the gut, making it both delicious and necessary for healthier food choices.

Kefir

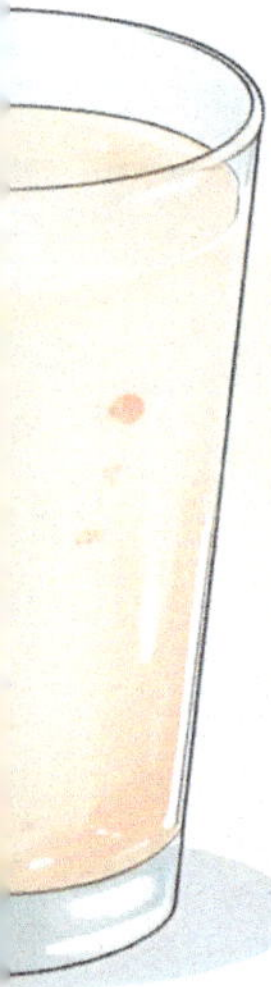

Kefir is an ancient fermented dairy product with a unique flavor and texture that was created in the Caucasus Mountains in Turkey. The process involves combining milk and sugared water with kefir grains, leaving a thinner version of yogurt. Kefir is rich in protein, calcium, probiotics, and B vitamins, supporting digestion, bone health, immunity, and overall well-being. It has up to 30 strains of probiotics and a wider variety of probiotic bacteria and yeasts than yogurt, making it a tiny ecosystem in a glass for a daily reset of your gut.

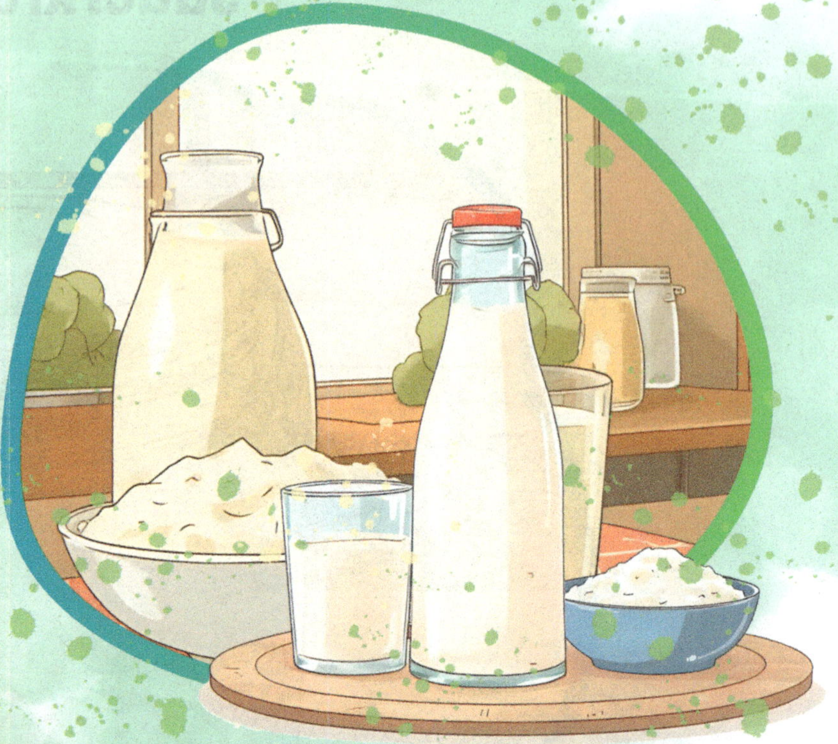

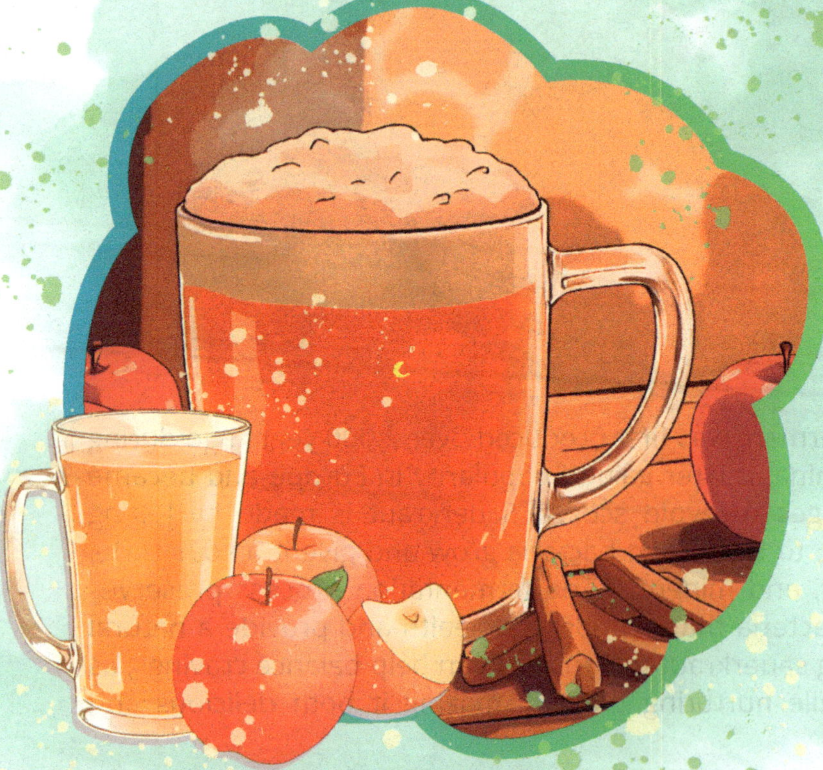

Apple Cider

Apple cider vinegar has a long history of use in both medicine and food preservation since the ancient Babylonians and Greeks. It is made from pressed fermented apple juice that is known for its richness in acetic acid, enzymes, potassium, and antioxidants. These nutrients help support digestion, balance blood sugar, boost metabolism, and promote healthy skin. Apple cider vinegar is often found in home kitchens and is readily available for use in home remedies for various common ailments, including wound care, cough relief, and stomach upset. Always dilute it in water to protect tooth enamel and avoid throat irritation.

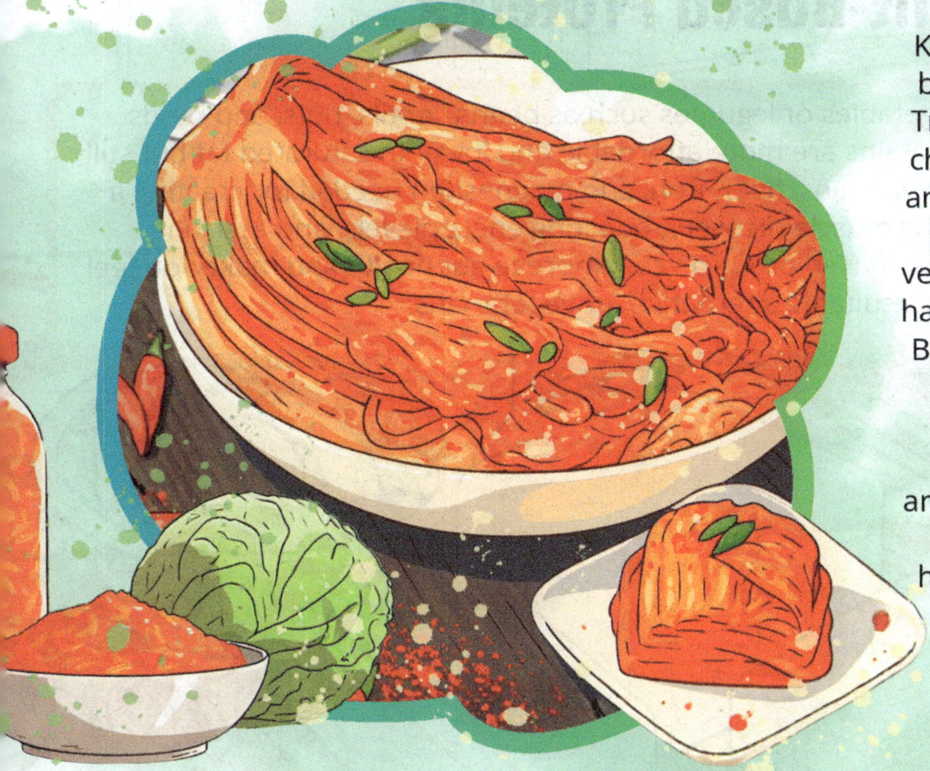

Kimchi

Kimchi is a popular Korean dish that has been around for more than 2,000 years. Traditionally, Napa Cabbage, radish, and chili were salted and seasoned with chili, and then fermented underground in clay pots called Onggi. This method allowed vegetables to ferment slowly through the harsh winter. Kimchi provides vitamins A, B, and C, along with beneficial probiotics that support gut health and immunity. The combination of spicy, tangy, and savory flavors makes it both delicious and with added probiotics. Aside from its nutritional value, it represents cultural heritage, family traditions, and seasonal harvests. In Korean culture, kimchi is a must-have at every meal

Miso

Miso has been around for more than a thousand years as food and valuable medicine. This traditional Japanese seasoning paste is made by fermenting soybeans with salt and koji mold over several months or even years to develop its complex flavors. This process creates a savory flavor called umami and adds depth to soups, sauces, and marinades. Miso is rich in protein, minerals, vitamins, and probiotics that are beneficial for the body and support gut health. Miso comes in various colors, flavors, and culinary grades, which are a favorite in many Japanese dishes. Even ancient Japanese monks ate miso to stay strong while fasting. Adding miso to your diet can make healthy eating feel indulgent.

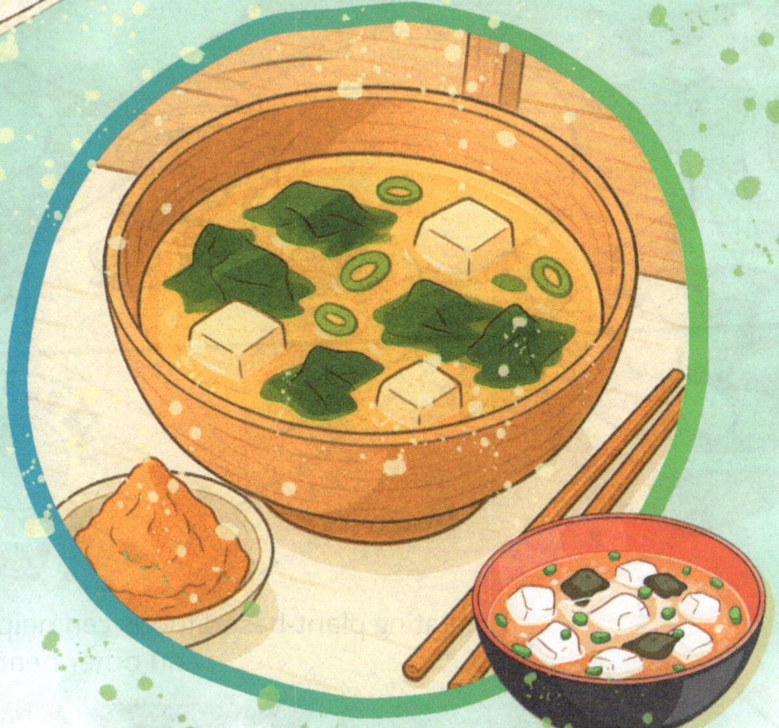

20. Plant-Based Proteins

Plant-based proteins come from vegetables or legumes such as beans, lentils, nuts, and seeds. Compared to animal sources, these proteins are more affordable and lower in saturated fat but still provide essential nutrients, including vitamins, fiber, iron, and magnesium needed for creating a strong and healthy physique, aiding muscle recovery, boosting energy levels, and assisting digestion. The high fiber content in plant-based products can improve gut health and make you feel fuller, making it a suitable alternative for vegetarians.

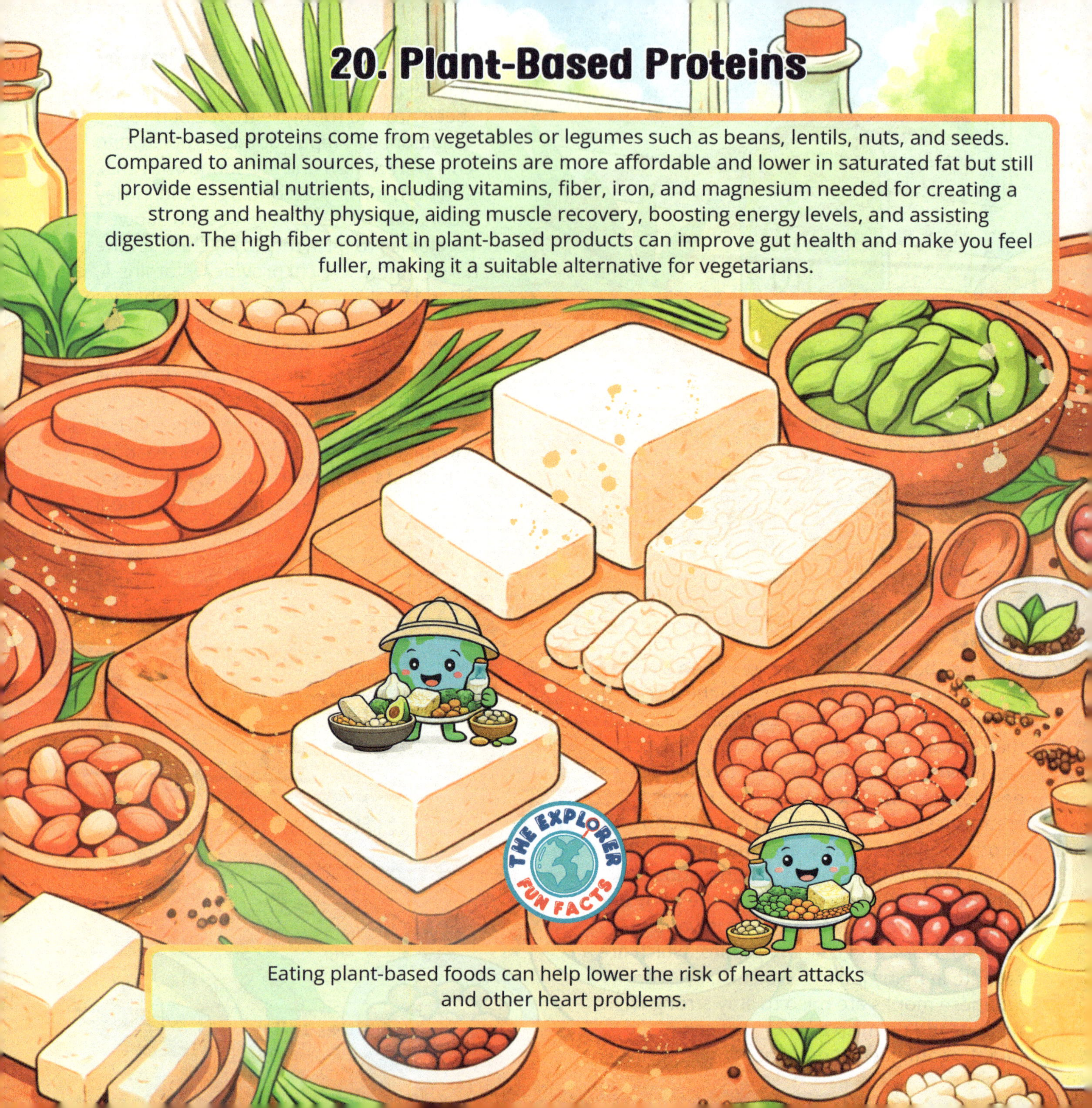

Eating plant-based foods can help lower the risk of heart attacks and other heart problems.

Tofu

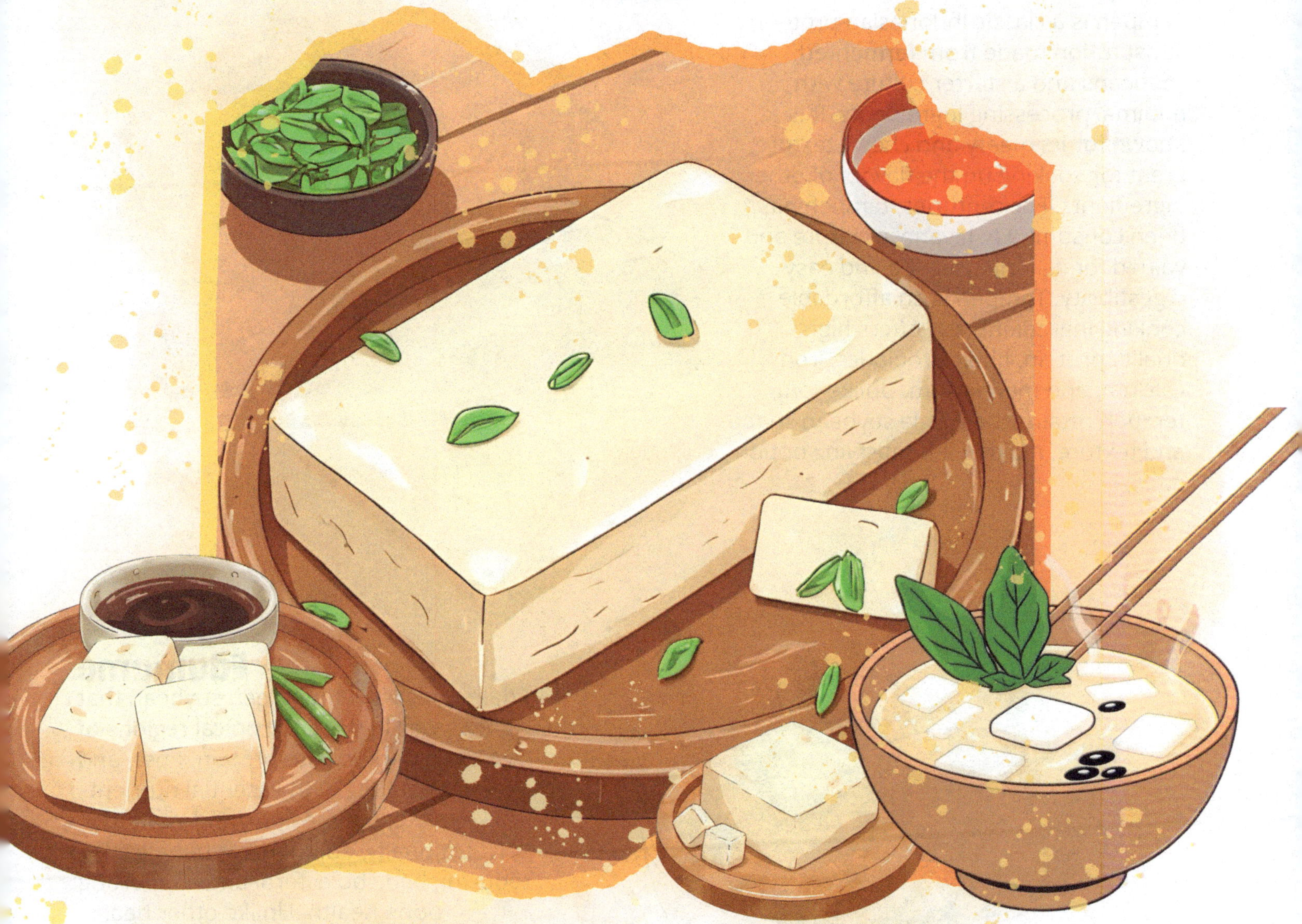

Tofu, made from soybeans, was accidentally invented in China about 2,000 years ago and has since become a popular food across Asia. Tofu has been a staple in Buddhist diets and traditions as a substitute for meat. It is made using a similar process to cheesemaking and pressed into a block, available in various firmnesses. Tofu has a creamy and slightly sweet taste from the soybean, absorb the flavors of any sauce or spice you cook it with. It provides protein, calcium, iron, and vital amino acids, and is praised for its quality in supporting balanced diets. It's a nutritious alternative for individuals seeking to build muscle without depending on animal products.

Tempeh

Tempeh is a classic Indonesian protein substitution made from fermented soybeans and a starter culture with minimal processing ingredients. It is known for its meaty and chewy texture, great for soaking up the flavors of other ingredients. For centuries, tempeh has been consumed in Javanese culture and valued for its long shelf life and easy digestibility. Tempeh is an affordable cooking ingredient that offers high quality protein, fiber, probiotics, iron, calcium, and magnesium. Unlike tofu, tempeh retains the whole soybean shape and texture, making it a satisfying option.

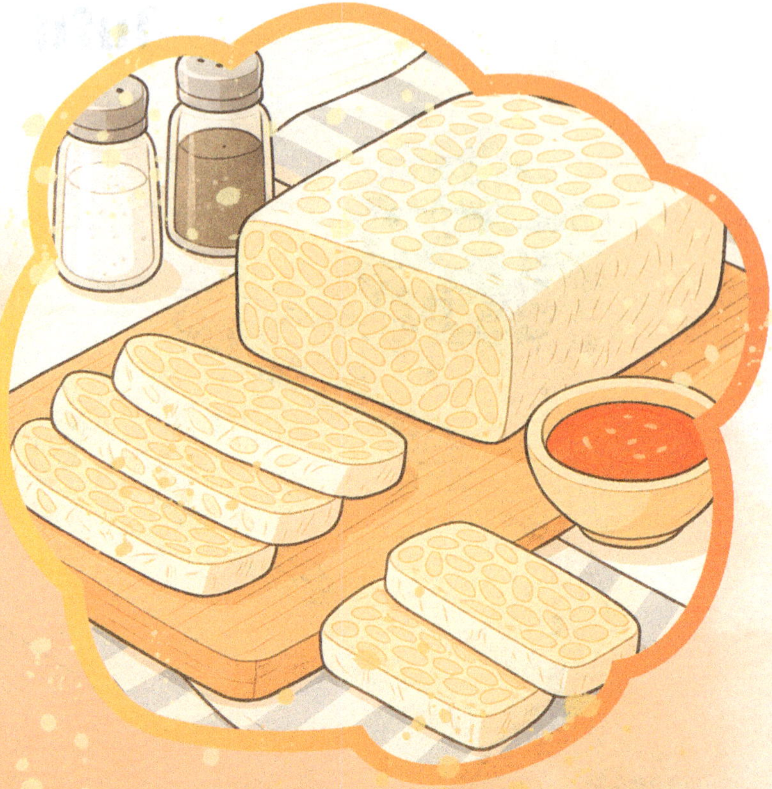

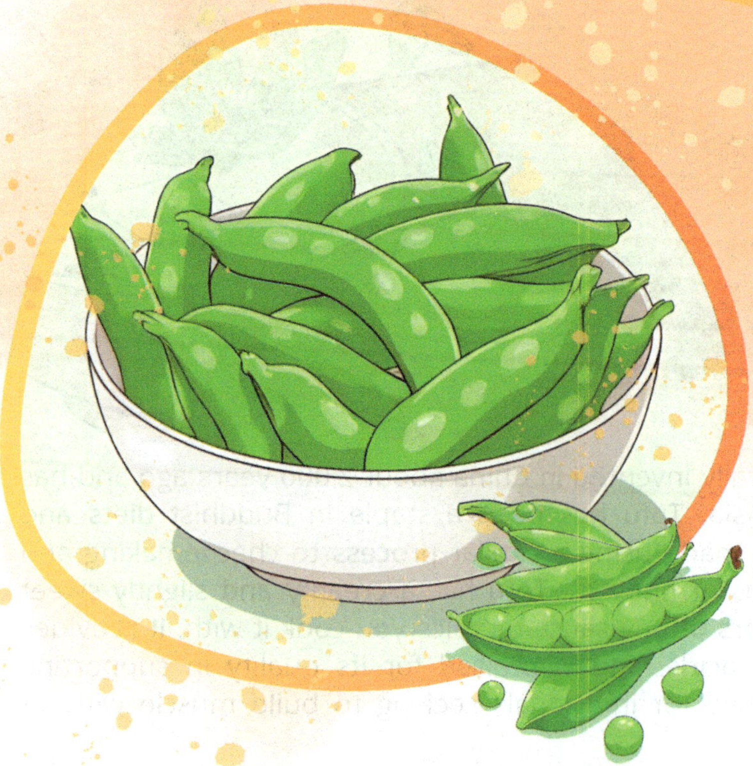

Edamame

Edamame is a young green soybean that grows well in the subtropical regions of Asia. It is packed with protein, fiber, and omega-3s, along with essential nutrients like folate, magnesium, and vitamin K. Nutritionally, edamame is beneficial in reducing bad cholesterol and supporting bone health. Unlike other beans, edamame offers complete protein that contains all the essential amino acids that the body cannot produce on its own. A single cup of edamame offers more protein than an egg, making it a healthy and tasty alternative that supports balanced diets.

Seitan

Seitan has been enjoyed in Asian cuisine for centuries, particularly among Buddhist communities in China and Japan. It is made by combining wheat gluten, extracted from wheat flour, with seasonings like nutritional yeast, paprika, garlic powder, and onion powder. The taste and texture offer a good protein content, and it delivers important minerals such as iron, calcium, phosphorus, and selenium. Remarkably, a single serving contains more protein than many animal meats, yet it is very low in fat, carbs, and cholesterol. Seitan is soy-free, making it an excellent option for those with soy sensitivities.

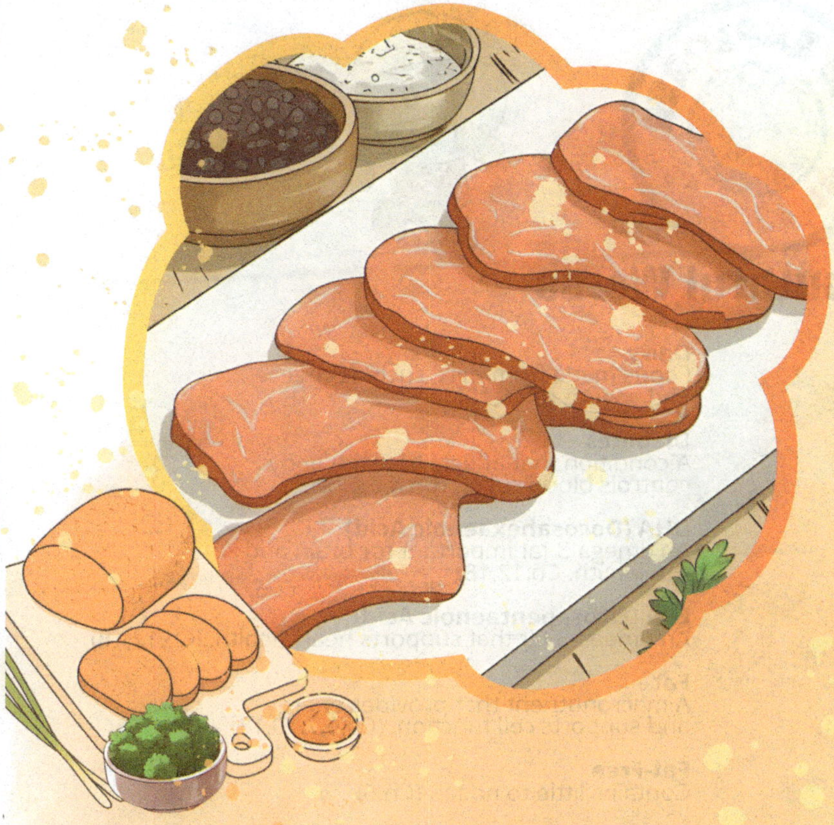

Lentil

The word lentil originates from the Latin word “lens,” which resembles its lens-shaped form. Lentils were first grown 8,000 years ago, and have been a food source since prehistoric times. Archaeologists discovered lentils buried in Egyptian tombs. Pharaohs believed they were food for the afterlife. As a cheap and simple ingredient to prepare, lentils are a dietary staple in Middle Eastern and Indian cooking. It is commonly added to soups, salads, stews, and curries. Lentils offer high amounts of protein, fiber, iron, and B vitamins. These nutrients improve digestion and help regulate energy.

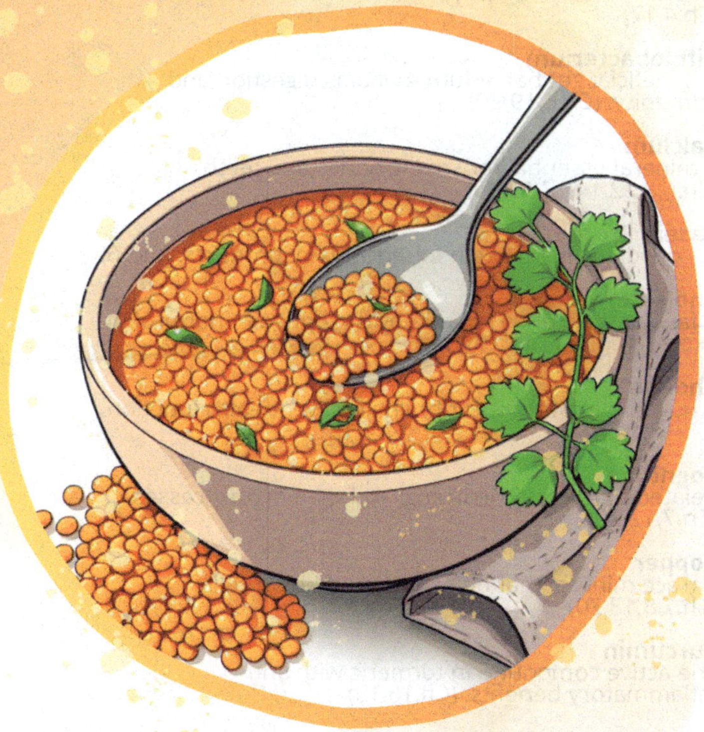

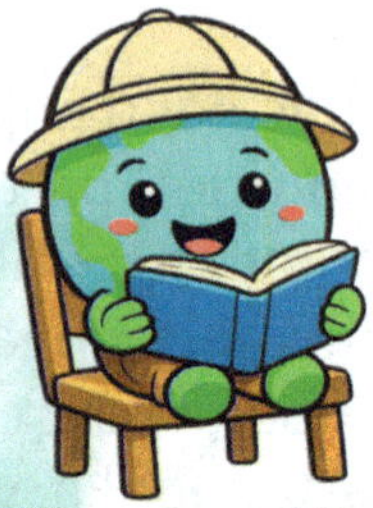

THE EXPLORER GLOSSARY

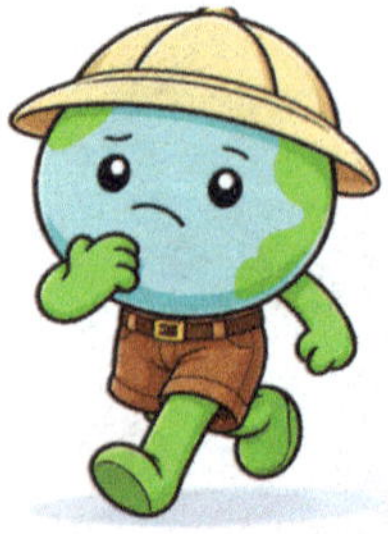

The Mouthful Words

Acetic Acid
A natural acid in vinegar that may help control blood sugar. (Ch.16,19)

Amino Acid
The building blocks of proteins are needed for growth and repair. (Ch.9,10,12,14,20)

Anemia
A condition where the body lacks enough healthy red blood cells. (Ch.10,17)

Antioxidant
A substance that protects cells from damage. (Ch.1,2,7,8,15,16,17,18,20)

Beta-glucan
A soluble fiber that supports heart and immune health. (Ch.4,17)

Bifidobacterium
A beneficial gut bacterium that aids digestion and immunity. (Ch.6,19,20)

Calcium
A mineral essential for strong bones and teeth. (Ch.6,8,12,14,17,19,20)

Casein Protein
A slow-digesting protein found in dairy products. (Ch. 6)

Cholesterol
A fat-like substance needed by the body but harmful in excess. (Ch.6,10,14,18)

Choline
A nutrient important for brain and liver health function. (Ch.12,14,20)

Cognitive
Related to thinking, learning, and memory processes. (Ch.7,12,20)

Copper
A trace mineral that helps form red blood cells. (Ch.7,8,13,20)

Curcumin
The active compound in turmeric with anti-inflammatory benefits. (Ch.16,19)

Dairy
Foods made from milk, such as cheese and yogurt. (Ch.6,19)

Diabetes
A condition that affects how the body controls blood sugar. (Ch.4,5,17)

DHA (Docosahexaenoic Acid)
An omega-3 fat important for brain and eye health. Ch.12,18)

EPA (Eicosapentaenoic Acid)
An omega-3 fat that supports heart health. (Ch.12,18)

Fat
A macronutrient that provides energy and supports cell function. (Ch.6,7,10,18)

Fat-Free
Contains little to no fat. (Ch.6)

Fiber
Plant material that supports digestion and the gut. (Ch.1,2,3,4,8,17,19,20)

Folate
A & B vitamin needed for cell growth and DNA formation. (Ch.2,3,8,17,18,20)

Fragariaphobia
An irrational and intense fear of strawberries. (Ch.1)

Glucose
A simple sugar and the main energy source for the body. (Ch.4,5,17)

Glycemic Index (GI)
A scale showing how fast foods raise blood sugar levels. (Ch.4,5,17)

Iodine
A mineral essential for thyroid hormone production. (Ch.12,20)

Iron
A mineral that carry oxygen in the blood. (Ch.2,3,10,11,13,17,20)

Isoflavones
Plant compounds with antioxidant and hormone-like effects. (Ch.3,20)

Lactic Acid
A substance produced during muscle activity and fermentation. (Ch.6,19)

Lactobacillus
A beneficial bacterium used in probiotics and fermented foods. (Ch.6,19,20)

Legume
A plant food such as beans or lentils rich in protein and fiber. (Ch.3,20)

Lectin
A protein found in plants that may affect digestion. (Ch.3)

Magnesium
A mineral involved in muscle, nerve, and energy functions. (Ch.4,7,8,17,20)

Manganese
A trace mineral that supports metabolism and bone health. (Ch.4,8,20)

Medium-Chain Triglycerides (MCTs)
Fats that are quickly absorbed and used for energy. (Ch.6,18)

Mercury
A heavy metal that can be toxic in high amounts. (Ch.12)

Metabolism
The process by which the body converts food into energy. Ch.4,5,7,17)

Microbiome
The community of microorganisms living in the gut. (Ch.6,19,20)

Mineral
Inorganic nutrients needed for body structure and function. (Ch 1-20)

Monounsaturated Fats
Healthy fats that support heart health. (Ch.7,8,12,18,20)

Myoglobin
A protein that stores oxygen in muscle tissue. (Ch.10)

Neanderthals
An extinct human species known for early dietary practices. Ch.12)

Neolithic Period
A historical era marked by farming and food domestication. Ch.4,20)

Niacin
A B vitamin important for energy metabolism. (Ch.4,10,12,20)

Omega-3 Fatty Acids
Healthy fats that support heart and brain health. Ch.12,18,20)

Parasite
An organism that lives off a host, sometimes causing disease. (Ch.10,12)

Phosphorus
A mineral important for bones, teeth, and energy production. (Ch.6,10,14,20)

Plant-Based Protein
Protein derived from plants such as legumes and grains. (Ch.3,4,8,20)

Porridge
A soft cereal dish made by boiling grains in liquid. (Ch.4,17)

Potassium
A mineral that helps regulate fluid balance and muscle function. (Ch.1,2,3,17,20)

Prebiotic
Fiber that feeds beneficial gut bacteria. (Ch.4,6,19)

Probiotic
Live beneficial bacteria that support gut health. (Ch.6,19,20)

Protein
A macronutrient needed for growth, repair, and enzymes. (Ch.3,9,10,12,14,20)

Rapid Eye Movement (REM)
A sleep stage associated with dreaming and memory. (Ch.9)

Resveratrol
A plant compound that helps protect against stress and damage. (Ch.1,17)

Riboflavin
A B vitamin important for energy production. (Ch.6,14,20)

Saturated Fat
A fat type that should be limited for heart health. (Ch.6,10,18)

Selenium
A trace mineral with antioxidant functions. (Ch.12,13,20)

Tryptophan
An amino acid involved in mood and sleep regulation. Ch.9,20)

Vegetarian
A diet that excludes meat and fish. (Ch.3,7,8,20)

Zinc
A mineral important for immunity and wound healing. (Ch.10,13,14,20)

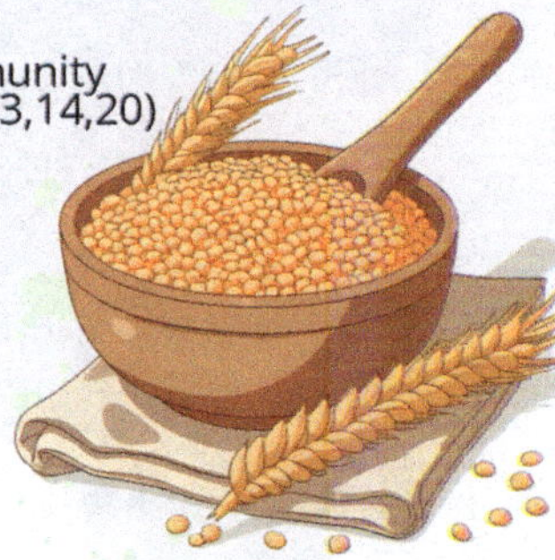

THE EXPLORER FUN FACTS

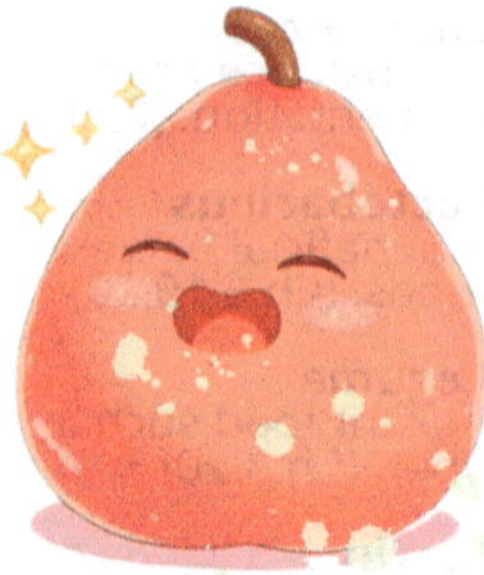

1.Did you remember what dry grape is called?
Raisin

2. What causes eye irritation and tears when chopping onions?
Onions take in sulfur from the ground while they're growing. When sulfur compounds mix with moisture in the atmosphere, they irritate the eye's nerves, resulting in tears.

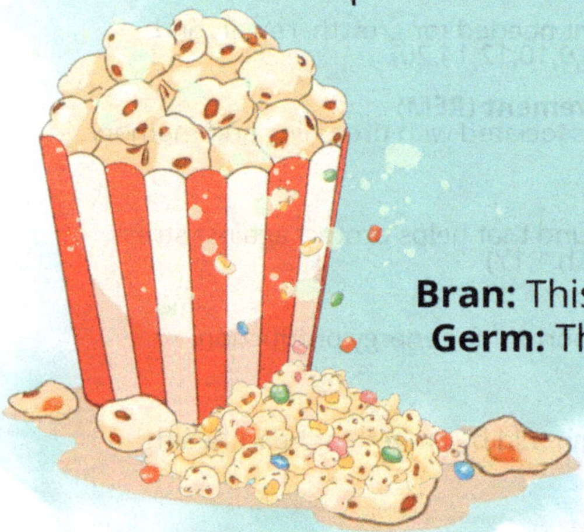

3. Is popcorn a bean or a whole grain?
Whole grain

4. What's Missing from Refined Grains?
Bran: This outer layer is full of fiber, which helps with digestion.
Germ: The tiny embryo of the grain, which contains important vitamins, minerals, and healthy fats.

5. How many layers are in refined grain?
A grain kernel has three parts: the bran (outer layer), the germ (the heart), and the endosperm (the starchy middle)

6. What is the red color in meat called?
The red color of meat comes from a blood protein called myoglobin that is responsible for storing and delivering oxygen to muscle cells during physical activity.

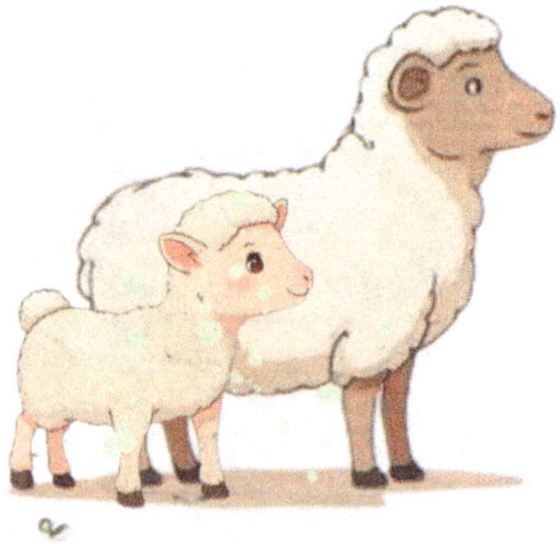

7. What is the unique thing about lambs?
Lambs have rectangular pupils that give 360-degree vision to spot predators and the ability to recognize their mother's sound as a way of communication.

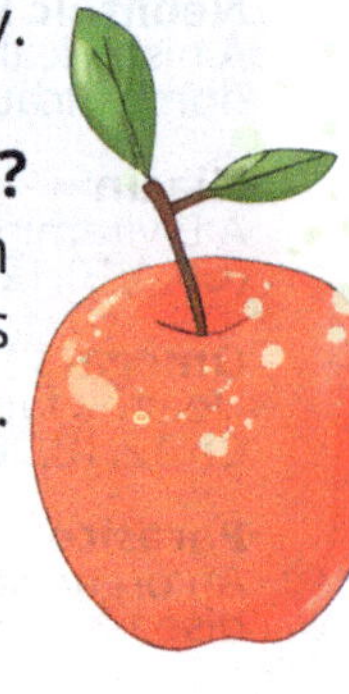

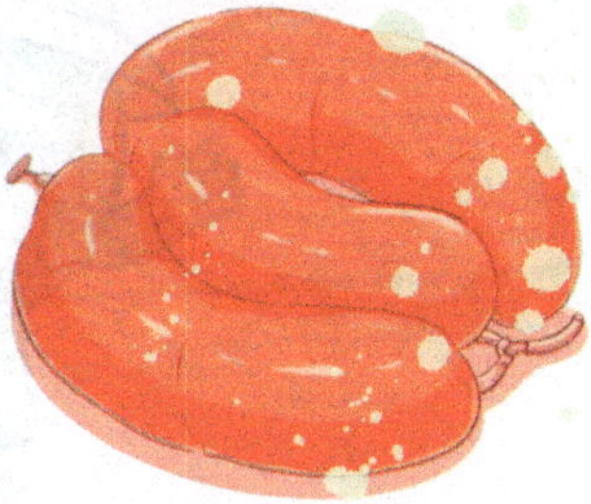

8. What are examples of food casing forms?
Some of the food casings used for sausages and hot dogs are mostly made from cleaned animal intestines of pigs, sheep, or cows.

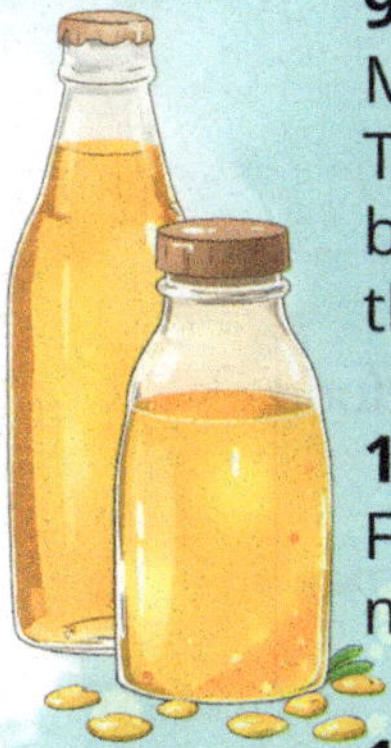

9. How many heart chambers do mammals have?
Mammals typically have four chambers in their hearts in total. The heart has two upper chambers that receive blood from the body and lungs. And two lower chambers that pump blood to the body and lungs.

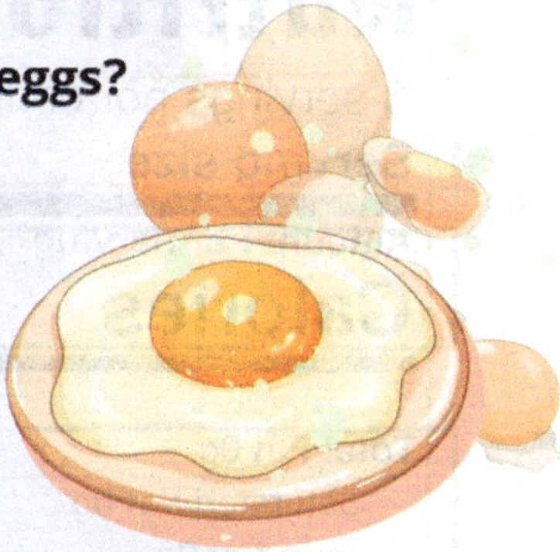

10. How can you tell the difference between fresh and old eggs?
Fresh eggs typically will sink. Likewise, the older eggs contain more air, causing them to float.

11. Why are healthy oils important for your brain?
About 60% of the brain is made of fat. Eating healthy oils gives the brain the best building block to improve memory and keep mind healthy and strong.

12. What are the "good" and "bad" bacteria living inside your body, and how can certain foods help the good ones?
Your body is home to trillions of bacteria. Nearly 85% are "good" bacteria that help with digestion, boost your immune system, and keep you healthy. The other 15% are "bad" bacteria that can make you sick. Eating fermented foods like yogurt, kimchi, or pickles helps good bacteria grow strong and keep harmful bacteria under control.

13. Which fruit actually has more potassium and fewer carbs than a banana?
It's the avocado! Avocados have more potassium, fewer carbs, lower sugar levels, and more fiber than bananas, making them a better choice for a healthy diet.

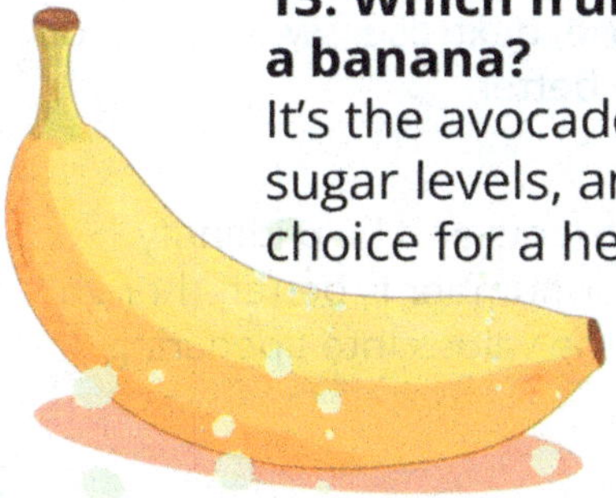

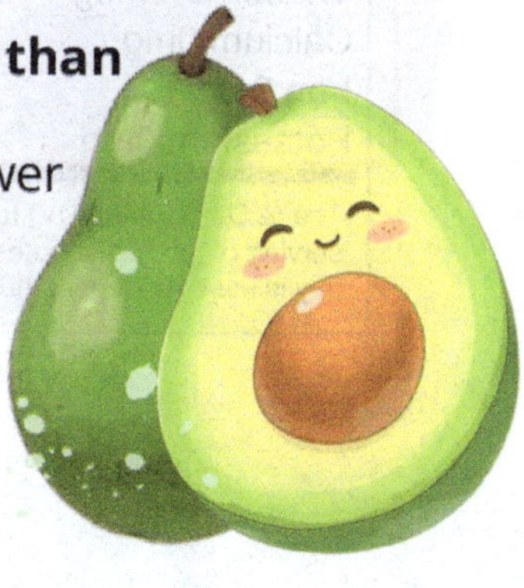

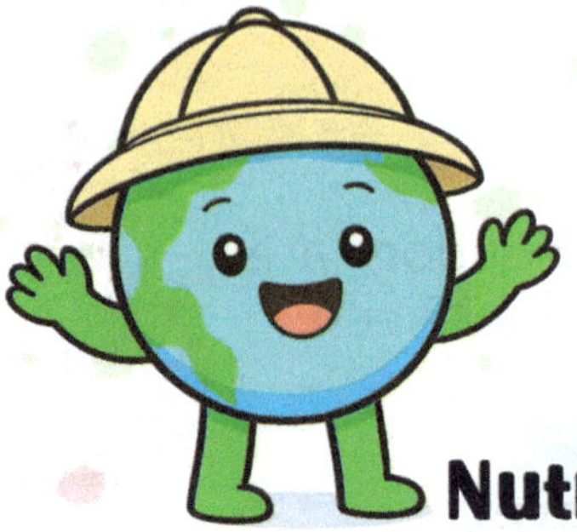

THE EXPLORER GUIDE

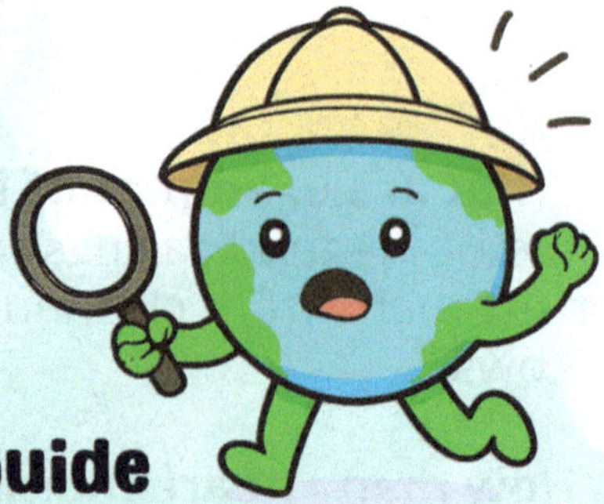

Nutritional Value Guide

How to read the Nutrition Facts (Kid Guide) label.

Nutrition Facts

5 servings per container

Serving size 1/2 cup (100ml)

Amount Per Serving

Calories 0

	% Daily Value*
Total Fat 0g	0%
Saturated Fat 0g	0%
Trans Fat 0g	
Cholesterol 0mg	0%
Sodium 0mg	0%
Total Carbohydrate 0g	0%
Dietary Fiber 0g	0%
Total Sugars 0g	
Includes 0g Added Sugars	0%
Protein 0g	0%
Vitamin D 0mcg	0%
Calcium 0mg	0%
Iron 0mg	0%
Potassium 0mg	0%

*The % Daily Value (DV) tells you how much a nutrient in a serving of food contributes to a daily diet. 2,000 calories a day is used for general nutrition advice.

① Serving size per container

Shows portion comparison of the amount of food you typically eat to the serving size listed.

② Calculated Calories Portion

Shows the number of calories per serving.

③ Percent Daily Values

Recommended nutrient goals or limits for a person. EX: 5% or less is low, 20% or more is high.

④ Fat & Sodium

Show quantity of saturated fat, trans fat, and sodium. Aim for low saturated fat. Watch out for foods with more than 20% of the DV of sodium. This indicates a highly processed food.

⑤ Dietary Fiber

A key to cancer prevention. Aim for foods high in fiber.

⑥ Sugar and Added Sugar

The amount of natural sugar from the product and the additional added sugar present in the product. Examples of added sugar include sucrose, dextrose, sweeteners, or honey. Less Added Sugar the better.

⑦ Vitamins & Nutrients

Represent essential micronutrients and help identify nutrient-dense foods. A higher number is better, though some junk food can mislead the values into appearing healthier.

The Explorer Selfie

Take a funny selfie of you and your favorite food's page.
Better yet, draw your favorite animal from this book here! Cheese!

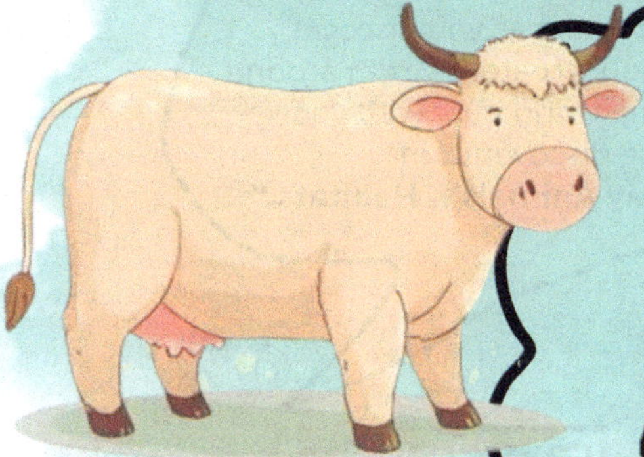

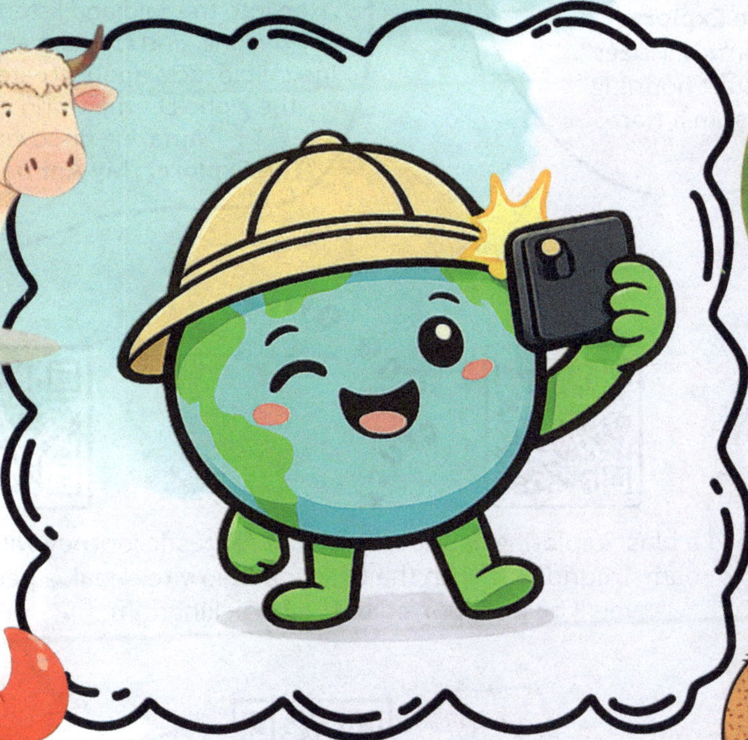

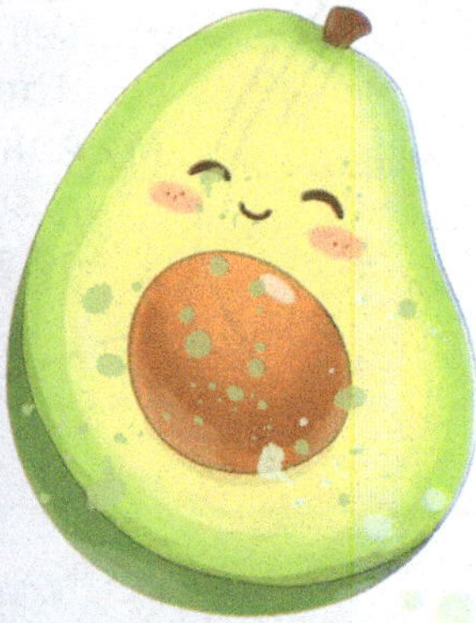

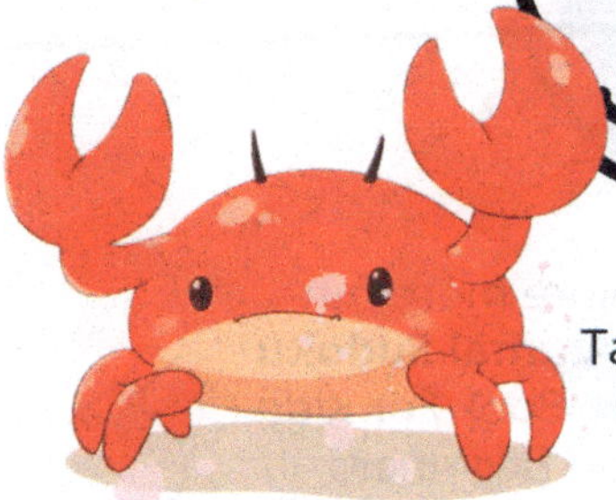

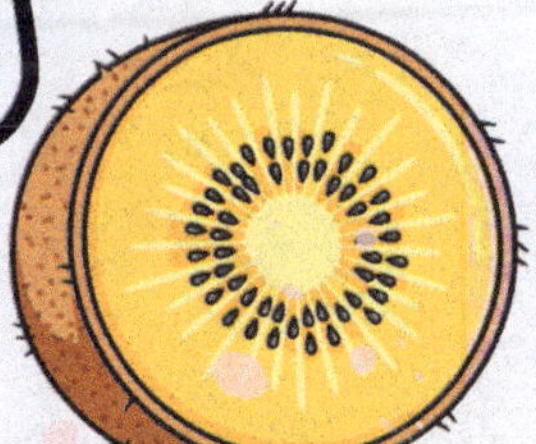

Snap and share!
Tag us your selfie or drawing on our social media
@liveandplaystudio
add hashtags
#liveandplaystudio #theexplorerfoodnutrition

THE EXPLORER INFO

Did you find where all the animals were hiding around the world? If that wasn't enough, get ready to A-MAZE yourself with over 100 **"The Explorer My Animals Mazes".** Yup, start hopping and scan it here!

You've traveled around the world munching on some of the most nutritious and delicious foods. Now, continue your adventure and explore the amazing world of animals and their habitats.
Hop into the wild and listen for the mooing, oinking, and clucking as you discover incredible facts about creatures from around the globe.Let the world buzz with your amazing discoveries in **"The Explorer: My Animals & Habitats."**

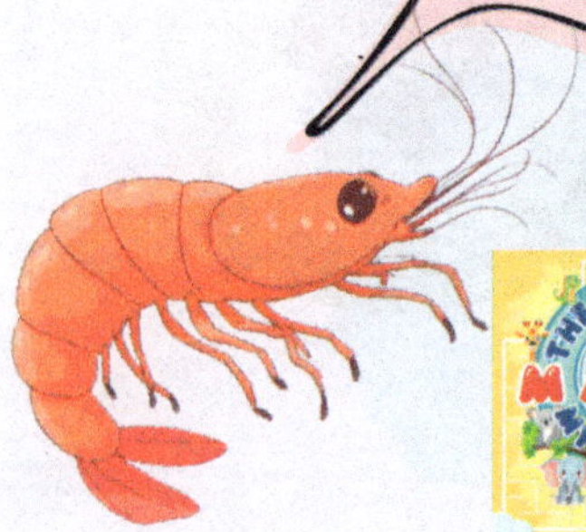

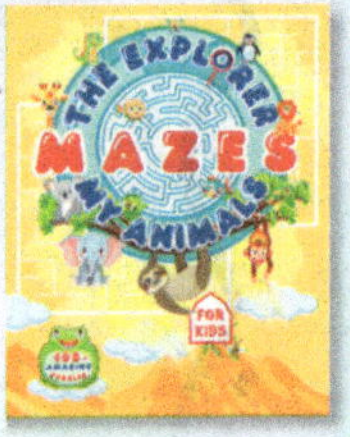

moo oink cluck

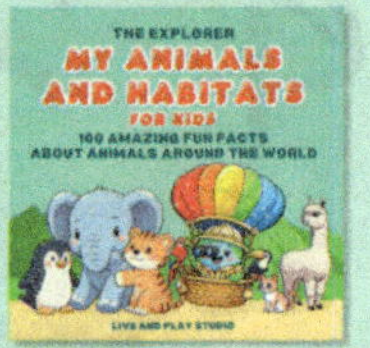

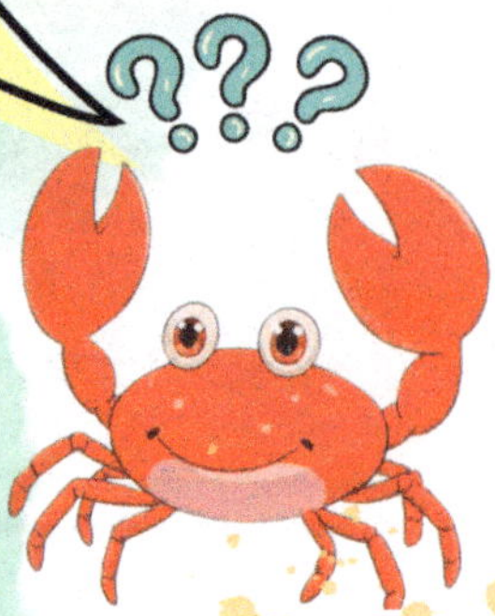

If you had a blast exploring, let's continue our fantastic journey with more books to roam around. Just scan the QR code below to sneak a peek, and you'll be transported to the book kingdom.

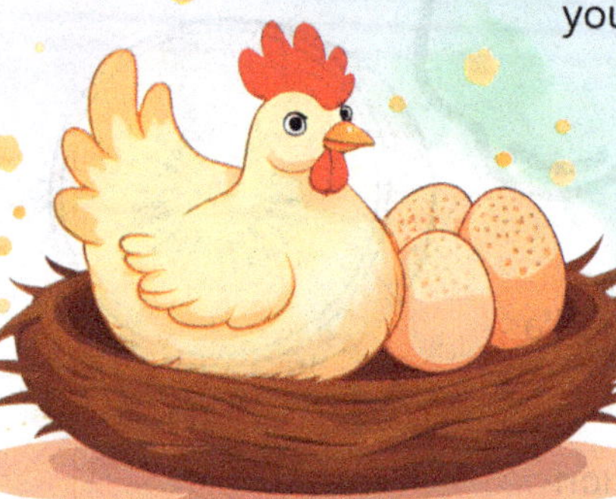

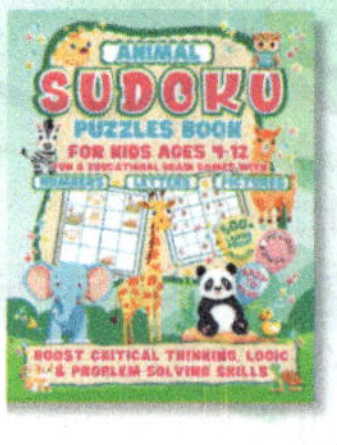

Explore more fun with **Animal Sudoku Puzzle** Book For Kids and Beginners

LIVE AND PLAY STUDIO

WWW.LIVEANDPLAYSTUDIO.COM

Continue your Food & Nutrition journey and unlock the best yet: **The Explorer Printable Bonus!** Get your **puzzles, recipes, journal, planner, and more.**
As our valued explorer, download this bonus for free by scanning the link below.

To instantly access your free **My Explorer printable**, simply scan the code below.
Start exploring new games and information right away!

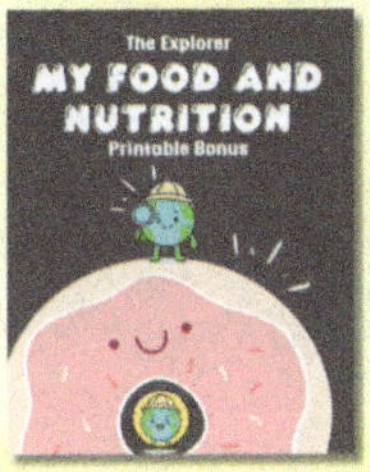

Free Printable
The Food Explorer Jounal

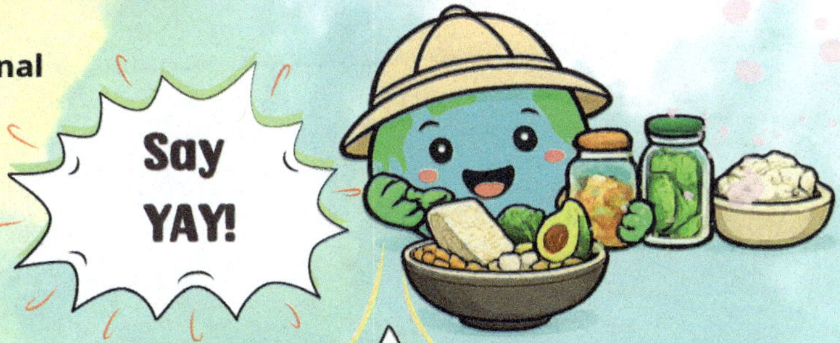

Thank you for choosing or book. Don't forget to sneak in or social media to catch up on more fun animations.

SCAN ME

REVIEW LINK

We would like to thank all of the fantastic readers who have purchased this book!

We sincerely hope this book has brought you joy, knowledge, and a world of imagination. As a small, independent publisher, your support means the world to us. If you can spare 60 seconds, we kindly ask you to leave your feedback and review to help us improve.
To do so, please scan the code below.

SCAN ME

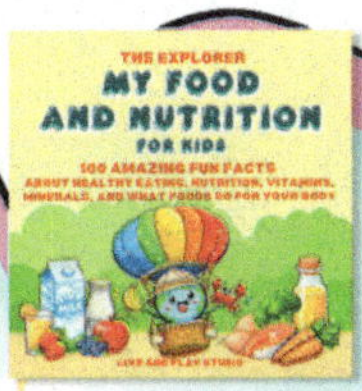

WWW.LIVEANDPLAYSTUDIO.COM

Made in the USA
Monee, IL
02 November 2026

67383580R00057